The Pare
Survival Guide to PANDAS/PANS

A Handbook to Manage Neuroimmune Disorders in Your Child Without Losing Your Mind

By

Deborah Marcus

Marcus, Deborah L

The Parent's Survival Guide to PANDAS/PANS: A Handbook to Manage Neuroimmune Disorders in Your Child Without Losing Your Mind / Deborah Marcus – 1st ed.

Includes bibliographical references and index.

ISBN: 9780578981642

This book is dedicated to my two daughters with PANDAS/PANS. Our journey together has helped me experience a level of patience, strength and love I never knew I was capable of. Thank you for allowing me to tell our story to help others.

I love you.

Contents

Introduction

In the summer of 2014, my younger daughter, then 6, began having extreme tantrums that were not age-appropriate. Soon after, she experienced stomach pains so intense she didn't want to eat. Then she had pain in one eye. The symptoms got progressively worse. In the process of trying to figure out what was causing her issues, my older daughter started exhibiting a few similar symptoms.

As we explored every avenue, my mother-in-law said she thought the ailments sounded similar to her friend's grandson, who had tickborne illnesses and PANDAS/PANS. Thankfully, our gastroenterologist was willing to test my younger daughter for Lyme disease while she was under anesthesia for an endoscopy. If it weren't for those two key pieces of the puzzle, I don't think we would have gotten answers so quickly. We got in touch with the parents of that grandchild, who educated us about tickborne illnesses and PANDAS/PANS and pointed us in the direction of an excellent LLMD (Lyme Literate Medical Doctor, a practitioner who treats Lyme disease and other co-infections). It took nearly a year and six physicians to get the proper diagnoses and uncover the root causes.

That year was a complete and utter nightmare for our whole family. It drained us physically and emotionally. It challenged our patience, strength and resilience. It tore us apart, yet we clung tightly to each other, as there was no one else to turn to. We all learned the definition of unconditional love. At that time, there was minimal support and virtually no mainstream understanding of PANDAS or PANS.

However, that year changed me for the better. It taught me to listen to my mama gut and trust my instincts. I discovered that my type-A personality was great for medical research but that I would need to let go of daily expectations if we were going to survive each and every day. My husband and I uncovered the true meaning of marriage – supporting each other through good times and bad – and how to lean on each other to weather the storm.

That was the hardest year of our lives, and we continue to face ups and downs as both of our girls still experience flares. However, I have realized it is time to pass on what I have learned over the past several years.

Until now, there have been very few books to help parents of PANDAS/PANS children navigate this difficult road on a day-to-day basis. I know I would have given anything for a survival guide to help me manage this challenging, confusing and isolating illness. So here I am, writing it for you, hoping to save you precious time, finite money and countless tears.

This book is designed to help you get through each day as you manage a child battling PANDAS or PANS. You can and you will. Let's face it: There is no choice. As you make your way through this guide, you will read stories that will help you realize that you are not alone. What you are going through is similar to what we and others have gone through.

Remind yourself that you are an amazing parent doing the absolute best you can for your child. On the toughest days, remember that you are enough. Be sure to look out for the silver linings along the way, as you will discover some.

As you learn through your own journey, please share your knowledge and support with others. Pay it forward. No one can or should face these disorders alone.

In this book, I have referred to a PANDAS/PANS child as "she" or "her." This was for the sole purpose of simplification. A child with PANDAS/PANS can be any gender with which one identifies.

I will share stories about "my daughter." While I have two daughters with PANDAS/PANS, I will intentionally not distinguish between them to respect their privacy.

For brevity, I'll refer to PANDAS/PANS as P/P for the rest of this guide. In cases where I need to specify which disorder I'm writing about, I will distinguish between the two.

Throughout this book, you will see the terms "flare" and "episode." A flare often refers to an extended period of time with increased symptoms, which can last days, weeks, months or years. A spike in behavior is often referred to as an episode. Some people will use these terms interchangeably, while others will refer to an episode as a reaction. Between episodes, the child is still in a flare.

This book was written during the first year of COVID-19; however, many of the stories take place prior to the pandemic, and the advice should be relevant regardless of the current state of the outbreak and well after the pandemic ends.

This book has been designed as your personal reference guide. Throw it in your bag and take it with you. Underline, highlight and circle information that resonates with you. Take notes and refer to them. Bring it to your physician and share it with your family and friends.

I am a mom, wife, daughter and friend. However, I am not a medical professional. This survival guide is designed to help you handle the P/P journey; however, it is not a substitute for a medical diagnosis and treatment from a licensed medical professional. This guide intentionally does not dive too deeply into diagnosis and treatment for that reason. This book does not have all the answers, as research continues to evolve, and the P/P community is learning more day by day. It should be used as a starting resource. If you suspect your child has P/P, I urge you to immediately seek out medical assistance.

Chapter 1: Symptoms of PANDAS and PANS

Before we dive into how to handle being the parent of a P/P child, let us first define what these illnesses are and what causes them.

According to PANDAS Network, a nonprofit organization dedicated to furthering research, treatment and support, the difference between PANDAS and PANS is the illness trigger.

PANDAS

PANDAS, an abbreviation for Pediatric Autoimmune Neuropsychiatric Disorders Associated with Streptococcal Infections, occurs when streptococcal (commonly known as "strep") triggers a misdirected immune response that results in inflammation of a child's brain.

When you hear the term "strep," it is often referred to as "strep throat," because it is commonly accompanied by a sore throat, white spots on the tonsils, and a fever. Other symptoms may include upset stomach, headache and more. Yet, it is incredibly important to know that strep is not limited to the throat. It can occur in the ears, in the sinuses, in the gut, on the skin, in the vagina, around the penis and in the area around the anus.

As a result, a traditional throat swab will not give you a positive result for strep when it is occurring somewhere else in the body. So, when exploring whether strep is your child's trigger, it is important to test beyond the throat. Also important to know is that the overnight strep culture test may show strep when the rapid test does not, so be sure to always request both.

My good college friend in Dallas has a daughter who had been exhibiting symptoms of P/P for a few years. For a while they chalked it up to her young age and then thought her restrictive eating was caused by an eating disorder. Her eating disorder diagnosis was reinforced by all of her doctors (including a pediatrician, gastroenterologist, therapist and psychologist). They were wrong. It was only one piece of the puzzle.

I encouraged my friend to get her daughter tested for strep throat. At the time, she was more focused on trying to get her daughter to eat for fear of malnutrition. She argued that her daughter did not have any symptoms of strep. But, at my urging and after reading some materials I had sent her, she told her daughter's pediatrician that strep was going around the classroom and asked to get her tested.

The pediatrician initially refused testing because there were no visible symptoms. My friend begged. When the test came back positive, she breathed a sigh of relief. The doctor was shocked. The pieces of the puzzle were slowly coming together. Strep can be present, even if you cannot see it, so do not rule it out without a test.

PANS

PANS, short for Pediatric Acute-onset Neuropsychiatric Syndrome, is thought to occur when an infection, virus, environmental factors or other possible triggers create a misdirected immune response, which results in inflammation of a child's brain. According to the PANDAS Network, children may experience symptoms after a "strong stimulant" to the immune system. In this case, it is not strep but could be Lyme disease or other tickborne illnesses (Bartonella, Babesiosis, Rickettsia, Ehrlichia, Anaplasma, etc.); mycoplasma pneumonia; Coxsackie (which causes hand, foot and mouth disease); MRSA (which causes a staph infection); other viral infections (including influenza and the common cold); Mast Cell Activation Syndrome (MCAS); allergens; yeast, mold or other toxins; or environmental triggers. Some parents believe they have observed PANS symptoms occurring after vaccine administration.

The research on PANS triggers has been limited, but it is evolving. In an effort to help better understand the root causes, Jessica Gavin, the founder of PANS Research and Advocacy Initiative (PRAI), launched the International PANS Registry in 2020. The goal was to gather data on P/P cases as a basis to advance research and shed light on the disease.

In discussing the rationale behind starting the study, Gavin said, "I started a group on Facebook asking questions and encouraging other PANDAS/PANS families to ask questions. The same questions were asked over and over again, like about mold, Lyme, dark circles under the eyes and ketosis pilaris. The commonalities were incredible, yet there was nothing in the literature. I really felt like the research was lacking. The question I asked of physicians was, 'What type of information would help convince you PANDAS/PANS is real?'"

Trying to get to the root cause of PANS in your child can be very challenging, as there is such a wide variety of illnesses that could cause it. However, knowing the potential causes will give you and your physician a place to start. We will explore this more in Chapter 2. Please note, this guide is not medical advice and not intended to help self-diagnosis. It is written to help provide you with the resources you need to get your child properly diagnosed and treated, and to help you manage P/P in your child, family and life.

Impact on the Brain

Without getting too technical, here is a basic explanation of how P/P affects the brain and body. Neurologists believe these illnesses affect the basal ganglia portion of the brain. The basal ganglia is located at the base of the forebrain and top of the midbrain. It is associated with a variety of functions, including control of voluntary motor movements, procedural learning (unconscious, long-term memory), habit learning (driven by a repetitive stimulus and response), eye movements, cognition and emotion. It is the section of the brain that is responsible for the body's fight-or-flight response.

In P/P, the receptors inside the basal ganglia are "attacked" by the immune system in an autoimmune fashion. For example, in an autoimmune thyroid condition, the immune system attacks the thyroid gland. In P/P, the immune system attacks this part of the brain.

Symptoms

Now that you understand how these illnesses may impact the basal ganglia portion of the brain, you will better understand the specific symptoms that are associated with these illnesses. These symptoms may come on rapidly and you may feel like they have come out of left field. One minute your child is fine and the next day she is a completely different person. The symptoms are severe and intense and can be incredibly hard to manage as a parent.

In Chapter 2, you will read about the criteria for a clinical diagnosis of PANDAS and PANS defined by the National Institute of Mental Health (NIMH). One of the key criteria listed is that the symptoms must have an acute onset. I want to underscore that these are the prevailing guidelines; however, not all parents experience their child's symptoms that way. In fact, some parents have reported that looking back, there were soft signs prior to the larger symptoms. For us, my daughters each had a dominant symptom at the start and then got additional symptoms later on.

It is important to note that a child can get both PANDAS and PANS. One of my daughters first had PANS due to Lyme and other tickborne illnesses. For a while she was feeling much better and off all medicine, only to catch strep throat and have a PANDAS flare.

Traditional P/P symptoms include, but are not limited to:

- Tics (involuntary sounds or spasm-like movements)
- Obsessive-Compulsive Disorder (OCD)
- Generalized anxiety

- Separation anxiety
- Restrictive eating
- Rage/aggressive behavior
- Oppositional defiance
- Hallucinations/intrusive thoughts
- Urinary issues
- Decline in math and handwriting abilities
- School refusal
- Personality changes
- Attention-deficit/hyperactivity disorder (ADHD)
- Sensory sensitivities
- Sleep disturbances
- Dilated pupils
- Dark rings under the eyes
- Pale skin

P/P symptoms may not all begin at once, and some children only have a few of these symptoms. If there is an underlying condition, you may see other bodily symptoms and ailments first. You might also question the more psychological symptoms that arise and wonder if they are age-appropriate or due to puberty.

Later in this book you'll hear from children themselves, in their own words, about how it feels to have this disorder. But for now, we're going to talk about each of the most common symptoms and how parents describe seeing them in their kids.

Tics

Tics can be vocal (humming, throat clearing, clicking one's tongue against the roof of the mouth, grunting or yelling out a word, for example) or motor (like blinking, shrugging shoulders, head twisting or mouth grimacing).

One of my daughters developed a tic where she would do a little body shake, like a shiver. At night, she would also feel the need to close her eyes tightly.

Another friend of mine in New York had a son who would touch his face repeatedly the same way thousands of times a day. Watching it drove her nuts. Eventually realizing he could not control it broke her heart.

One mom from Iowa shared that her son would "lift his shoulders to his ears, tuck his elbows to his ribs and then bring his hands up to the front of his face and wiggle his fingers. We called them butterfly fingers because we didn't know that it was a tic," she said. "We just knew that he did it when he was agitated, bored or excited. It might go away for a few days but would keep coming back."

Another friend noticed early on that her son would open his mouth wide, almost like he was stretching his face, several times a day. It wasn't super noticeable and it was the only tic he ever had. His other symptoms, including rage, OCD and oppositional behavior, were much more debilitating. The tic eventually went away as he healed.

One PANDAS parent from Texas noticed her daughter would clear her throat. While clearing one's throat is common, the thing that made it a tic was the repetitive nature of it. Many parents may have overlooked it.

OCD

Sometimes anxiety and obsessive-compulsive disorder can be difficult to distinguish between. Dr. Deborah Glasofer, an assistant professor of clinical psychology, says that while people with anxiety tend to worry a lot, they don't tend to engage in ritualistic behaviors to cope with their anxiety.[1] "People with OCD, however, commonly use repetitive behaviors – either physical or mental rituals called compulsions – to relieve the stress caused by an obsession," she said.

OCD was a huge symptom for both of my children. Normally, they would fixate on one thing for a week or two and then it would pass, and they would be on to the next fixation. The fixations were bizarre, to say the least, and drove us all a bit crazy.

One week, the door to my daughter's room had to be open just the right amount. Not too much. Not too little. I

---

[1] www.verywellmind.com/what-is-the-difference-between-gad-and-ocd-1393010

spent easily an hour adjusting and readjusting the door position while she cried and screamed. The OCD was torturing her.

During another P/P flare caused by Lyme, my daughter would not leave the bathroom for hours. At first, she was using the toilet frequently due to stomach pain, but even as she healed, it turned into OCD. It got to the point where she was unable to attend school for a few weeks. She would sit on the toilet while doing homework on a tray table. I would sit on a stepstool beside her. Eventually, we got through it.

Many parents share that their P/P children are germophobic. A good friend had a daughter who feared her sister for a long time because she thought she was "germ infested." Strangely, this fear did not extend to her parents. As part of this fear of germs, her daughter would take five showers a day. While the water bill was high, it did calm her in the moment.

Similarly, another boy would wash his hands a lot and obsess over anything touching his lips. Even if nothing really touched his lips, he would cry and insist that it did.

One parent said her child would need to repeat things over and over until he was satisfied with the way it sounded. Another needed to give a play-by-play of everything he was doing the entire time he was doing it. For example, if he was playing with a puzzle, he would say, "I'm doing a puzzle. I'm doing a puzzle. I'm doing a puzzle." Another child would tell his mother what he was doing and insist that she tell the dog everything, even if the dog was nowhere in sight.

A parent in Texas spent months wondering whether her son had P/P. Though her 9-year-old had almost every other symptom, she was confused because he didn't seem to have any OCD symptoms. Later she realized that OCD just looked different in her son.

At the onset of P/P, he had suddenly refused to brush his teeth. He then refused to take baths, raging at the mention of it. Occasionally, when he could get in the bath, he would tell her he couldn't get out, sitting helplessly in the bath for up to a half-hour longer. He would never say why he couldn't brush his teeth or get out of the bath; when he started to open up about it months later, he would only say, "I feel like I'm going to die."

He would also get ideas, like suddenly wanting to rearrange the furniture in his room at midnight, and then could not get the idea out of his head. He would begin to rage if his parents told him no. It wasn't simply a kid not getting his way; my friend could see that once her son had something in his head that "had" to happen, absolutely nothing else would do.

Anxiety

The anxiety is also incredibly debilitating. My daughter would be preoccupied with one thought that would take over and not allow her to think rationally or clearly about things. For example, if she had one bad night's rest, she would be anxious about the next night's rest, convincing herself that she could no longer sleep. She would get upset about it for hours. Thank goodness we had a few tricks up our sleeves and great medical advice to help her fall asleep and break that cycle.

Specifically, separation anxiety and school anxiety are also common. My mother and aunt came to visit and watch the girls for a few hours so I could get a much-needed break while my husband was away on a business trip. My daughter would not let go of me when I tried to leave. She clung to me, hysterically screaming and crying as I slowly tried to calm her and peel her arm off my body. Eventually, I made it out the door. Keep in mind, this is a girl who, prior to P/P, would give me a hug and a kiss and say, "See you later."

Many parents reported that their once independent children who happily went to school before P/P, would suffer so greatly from anxiety that they were not able to attend school. There are examples from the children themselves later in this book.

Restrictive Eating

Restrictive eating is reported by many P/P parents. ARFID (Avoidant Restrictive Food Intake Disorder) is an example of this symptom. According to the National Eating Disorders Association, ARFID is similar to anorexia in that both disorders involve limitations in the amount and/or types of food consumed, but unlike anorexia, ARFID does not involve any distress about body shape or size, or fears of being overweight. Sometimes the child might be worried about the sensory characteristic of a food (the sensation of chewing or the feeling of swallowing), or they might be worried about throwing up after eating. Sometimes kids will slowly drop one food at a time from their list of "safe" foods.

One parent reported that their child was afraid of choking and would only eat vanilla ice cream and popsicles. Another child had an irrational fear of vomiting. She didn't feel nauseous, just scared that she might.

Other children may not eat because of stomach pain in combination of a fear of vomiting. This, in turn, may create more stomach pain due to hunger and become a vicious cycle. This can have dangerous implications.

PANDAS Physicians Network provides additional reasons for children with P/P not eating normally or adequately, including sensitivity to taste, smell and texture, fear that food has spoiled, or fear of being poisoned. The fear of being poisoned can also appear when a child refuses to take medicine.

Rage/Aggressive Behavior

Of all the symptoms, rage was probably the scariest. My husband and I felt like we were walking on eggshells, never quite knowing what would set our daughter off on a violent tantrum. Once she was in it, it was as if she was possessed. Her eyes would be dilated and opened wide. She would hit, scratch and bite anyone in her path. She would lay on the floor kicking and screaming. This would go on for hours if I did not interject, and I was the only one who could stop it, not my husband.

I would have to roll her on her back, lay my entire body weight on her, hold her arms down and softly whisper "shhh" in her ear until she calmed down. After she came out of her trance, she would sometimes go about her business as if nothing had happened at all. Sometimes she didn't even remember the episode.

One mom said that her son once threw a tantrum out of the house for a couple of hours and after the ibuprofen kicked in, he sat up and asked, "Why are we here?" Forgetting that an episode happened is more common than one might expect.

Some parents reported that their children's episodes would happen in a cycle. "His eyes would be big. He would be manic for 10 to 15 minutes, even laughing uncontrollably, and then raging for 30 to 40 minutes, and then hysterically crying for 15 minutes. After all this, he would crash for a half-hour. He would rapidly cycle through this."

Another P/P mom told me that her son's rages got so bad that she would walk around the house nauseous because she never knew what would set him off next. One time her husband went to the store to get ribs, but they were out of them. Her son was set on having ribs that night, and when his dad returned without them, he violently raged, locking his dad out of the house and demanding he get ribs somewhere, anywhere. He would throw their furniture over, break their TV and flip over their mattress. She said the things that set him off would sound ludicrous to outsiders.

At times, her husband would have to hold him down to keep the rest of the family safe. Her son would then go from rage-filled to panic-filled, screaming that his dad was trying to hurt him, or worse. His reaction was as if his dad was holding him down for no reason.

After each episode, he would be calm and remorseful, wanting to cuddle with them and be comforted. Months later, when his parents mentioned the ribs incident, he had no idea what they were talking about. He would rarely remember the episodes, even the next day. Eventually, with the right treatment, his rages disappeared.

Hallucinations/Intrusive Thoughts

According to Rethink Mental Illness, a hallucination is when you might see, hear, taste, smell or feel something that exists only in your mind. While my children never experienced hallucinations, many other children do.

One mom recalled an incident when her son was screaming at the pediatrician's office for her to sit in the chair and pick her feet up off the floor because there were snakes all over that were going to come and get them. The doctor, who was not educated on P/P, looked at the mom and said, "You can't make this up. If you told me that he did this at home, I wouldn't have believed you."

On a Facebook page for P/P, a mom shared that her daughter hallucinates. One time, her daughter went to sports practice and was laughing uncontrollably and thinking that her teammates' shirts reminded her of God, Jesus and the devil. Then, her eyes rolled back into her head and she fell.

Another mom said that during a hallucination, her son was hysterically screaming about thorns in his pants and was scratching his skin raw and ripping off his clothes. The mom checked; there was nothing there.

Hallucinations can be scary and confusing for the child, as well as the parent. Hearing voices, which is considered an "auditory hallucination," is different than an intrusive thought, which is defined by Rethink Mental Illness as "an unwelcome thought or image that enters your mind and is mostly out of your control. It won't sound as though others can hear it. It may be a disturbing thought such as harming people that you love."

Intrusive thoughts are also a common symptom among P/P children. For example, a parent said that her son has a fear or image that she will die, or he will kill her. This intrusive thought is sadly reported as common among the P/P community.

One 9-year-old with P/P kept thinking that all the trees are going to suddenly die, and the oxygen will disappear. Another intrusive thought he had was that gravity would stop and everyone would float away.

Urinary Issues

Often, children with P/P will experience urinary issues, which can take different forms. For one child it may be constantly feeling wet in the vaginal area, which results in excessive wiping and a very red, sore area.

For my daughter, it was the feeling of needing to go to the bathroom every five minutes, especially at nighttime (known as enuresis). It was so frustrating for her because she would be tired and ready to go to sleep, but would keep having to get up to urinate.

Other parents said that their previously potty-trained children suddenly start having accidents. One parent shared that during a flare her 7-year-old was having nightly bed wetting and even daytime accidents, which he hadn't had for years.

Handwriting & Math Issues

While the brain is under attack with P/P, many children experience issues with writing and math. Dysgraphia is common among children with P/P. According to *ADDitude* magazine online, dysgraphia is a "neurological disorder of written expression that impairs writing ability and fine motor skills," and "it interferes with practically all aspects of the writing process, including spelling, legibility, word spacing and sizing, and expression." In addition, OCD can be manifested as perfectionism. As a result, not only can a child have difficulty thinking creatively and writing out their ideas, once they do, they find themselves erasing and re-writing due to a desire for it to be perfect.

My daughter often wrote very small and lightly with her pencil. Her teacher could barely read it and complained that she needed a magnifying glass. We suspect this handwriting style was due to dysgraphia as well as sensory issues. When my daughter tried pressing harder on the pencil, she would then get frustrated by how messy it was and would erase repeatedly until there were holes in the paper. It was very frustrating all around.

Math skills often also become an issue with P/P. First, the child has challenges paying attention, poor short-term memory, reduced working memory and difficulty holding information. In addition, critical skills for implementing math concepts, such as planning and prioritizing steps, are also impacted. As a result, learning new math concepts and executing them becomes incredibly difficult.

My daughter was a straight-A student prior to P/P. When she entered a flare after a few years of her illnesses being dormant, her academic performance plummeted overnight. She started failing quizzes and exams. Math concepts became confusing and hard to remember. Sadly, this is all too common among children experiencing P/P. You will find additional examples in Chapter 5: The Child's Perspective.

Eyes & Skin

As you can see, most of the examples of symptoms provided in this chapter occurred in homes. Most family and friends never saw my kids this way and were somewhat shocked to hear that our daughters were sick because they looked just fine to them. If you looked closely at my girls, you'd notice dark circles under their eyes and paler skin than normal. In addition, during a rage or episode, their pupils would dilate. Some children with PANDAS experience peeling skin on the hands or feet, which are physical signs of strep. These are subtle but common symptoms among P/P children.

Prevalence Statistics

While you may feel like this illness is rare, it is estimated to affect 1 in 200 children, according to the PANDAS Network. It is more likely to affect boys than girls (2.6:1)[2]. Based on PANDAS Network research, among 700 self-reports, approximately 69% of P/P onset occurs among children ages 4-9 years old and 19% among children 10-13 years old. Nearly 11% is among children 1-3 years old and only 1% are ages 14+.

Later in this handbook, I will help you identify where to find other parents of P/P children so that you can develop a support system to help get you through this difficult time.

The resource section of this survival guide provides recommendations on websites, books, documentaries and more where you can get additional detailed and scientific information. I encourage you to explore these resources so that you may become a better advocate for your child.

---

[2] www.pandasnetwork.org/statistics/

Chapter 2: Diagnosis

If your child has already received a diagnosis of PANDAS or PANS, you have already overcome a big hurdle that many parents face. If you have not yet received the diagnosis, this chapter is intended to help you get there more smoothly.

When your child starts to exhibit P/P symptoms, you may not see them all at once nor put them all together. With children, it can be hard to decipher between what is an ailment worth paying attention to versus one that is just in the moment. It can also be difficult to determine if a behavior is age-appropriate or out of the norm.

In addition, you may find that your child's behaviors are different when at home versus outside the home. Your home is a safe space, so children tend to hold it together more in public and then break down at home. On the one hand, this can minimize scenes in public, but on the other hand your friends and family may not see what you see behind closed doors and may be skeptical that there is even an illness at play.

While the trademark trait for P/P is a sudden, acute and debilitating onset of symptoms, it is not always the case. As mentioned in Chapter 1, some children may change literally overnight, waking up one day with symptoms never seen before, while others experience changes more slowly. Therefore, I would urge you to ensure you are working with a physician who will not use this single criterion as the sole determining factor for diagnosis.

When my daughter first fell ill, she experienced stomach pains that got progressively worse. Then began pain in one eye followed by severely defiant behavior. This occurred over a few months. We saw her pediatrician, who didn't look at those symptoms as possibly connected; she was simply not capable, due to her lack of knowledge and understanding of P/P. She sent us to a gastroenterologist for her stomach issues and an ophthalmologist for her eye pain. We chalked up the challenging behavior to other situational changes going on at the time.

My mother, in an attempt to help, suggested that perhaps I was coddling her too much and not being strict enough with her behavior. Thinking her poor behavior was due to my lack of parental involvement or my parenting style could not have been further from the truth. My mother now knows otherwise.

The ophthalmologist did not see anything wrong with her eye. The gastroenterologist did an endoscopy and partial colonoscopy that only revealed general inflammation. It was the eventual inconclusive Lyme test and a visit with an LLMD, who was also well-versed in P/P, that ultimately resulted in a proper diagnosis, nearly a year later.

Unfortunately, while there have been advances in P/P research and awareness, there is still a long way to go to establish it within the medical community. There are still many doctors who do not believe in nor treat P/P. It can be an uphill battle trying to convince one of these doctors to believe that your child may have it.

Given how telemedicine has become more common and accepted, it may be easier than ever to find and meet with a knowledgeable P/P practitioner. Some doctors may require an initial in-person appointment and then allow virtual follow-up appointments for up to a year.

Remember, you know your child best, so trust your gut if something is not right. You are your child's best advocate. Do not give up until you get some answers. No one will fight harder for a proper diagnosis.

There are two things you can do to ensure you get an accurate diagnosis: symptom journaling and selecting the right physician.

Symptom Journaling

To create a symptom journal, I recommend purchasing an inexpensive notebook and writing down all the symptoms you observe with dates and times. Is she doing the same movement repeatedly? Is she excessively obsessing over situations or things? Write down related notes at the time as well. What did she just eat? Did she sleep enough last night? Is a certain piece of clothing bothering her? These will help you determine patterns and triggers.

Here are the most common symptoms to observe and track:

- Tics
- Obsessive-compulsive disorder (OCD)
- Anxiety/separation anxiety
- School refusal
- Personality changes
- Severe oppositional defiance
- Rage/irritability/aggressive behavior
- Attention-deficit/hyperactivity disorder (ADHD)
- Decline in math skills
- Decline in handwriting abilities
- Sensory sensitivities
- Sleep disturbances
- Restrictive eating
- Hallucinations/intrusive thoughts

- Urinary issues
- Dilated pupils
- Dark rings under the eyes

Be sure to take videos and pictures. When my daughter was in a P/P rage, which was completely inappropriate for her age, and included hitting, scratching and biting me, my husband videotaped it. It may sound cruel to videotape our child's worst moments; however, that proof helped the doctor see what was going on at home, which was not visible in the doctor's office.

When you visit the practitioner, you can bring the same notebook with you and use it to take notes at each appointment. It will also be helpful to keep track of medicine dosages and possible reactions. As you begin treatment, the notebook will help you keep track of whether symptoms are getting better or worse. This will keep all your child's illness records in one place. Even if it ends up not being P/P, you will still have a recorded history to uncover other possible illnesses.

Another piece of the puzzle that will be helpful to get the right diagnosis is a timeline of events. When did you first see symptoms? Was the child recently treated for strep throat or another illness? If so, for how long and with what medicine? Did she recently have a high fever or strange rash? Did you recently go camping and did your child wear bug spray? Was your child in tall grasses recently? Creating a timeline with dates and activities will help uncover the mystery.

Also consider your environment. Did you recently move into a new house? Did your child start attending a new school? Think about the condition of the places your child is spending her time. Is the building old or new? Is there any indication of water damage, mold or toxins? Does your child seem to do better or worse when she is away from the house for a few days?

"Parents who keep a timeline and notebook of events to share with their provider have been so helpful," said Jana Roso, who treats many P/P kids at her practice, Alive and Well in Austin, Texas.

Selecting a Practitioner

The next most important step is to find the right doctor or practitioner – one who believes in and has experience treating P/P. You want to find a specialist who will listen to you. As we will discuss later in this chapter, P/P requires a clinical diagnosis, so your journal with examples of symptoms will be critical to ensure a proper diagnosis.

There are a few different resources to explore when searching out a specialist near you. PANDAS Physicians Network has a searchable database of practitioners. There are also quite a few P/P groups on Facebook, nationally and state-specific, where individuals may recommend practitioners near you who they have experience with. The resource section of this survival guide will provide contact information for these Facebook groups.

Lastly, you may want to reach out to others and ask around. You might be surprised to know that a friend of a friend is a P/P parent and can point you in the right direction.

Many P/P physicians charge a hefty fee upfront (several hundred dollars to more than $1,000), as they need to spend a lengthy amount of time with you and your family to evaluate and diagnose. Also, in some states, these physicians do not take insurance. If you can afford it, I highly recommend spending the money upfront to see a specialist with experience. Getting a proper diagnosis and beginning treatment as soon as possible is the key to getting it resolved more quickly.

While you may start with your pediatrician, they may not be as educated as you are on the subject. You may encounter physicians who don't believe in P/P and it can be quite a challenge to convince them.

A mom from Iowa shared the following story: "When I took my son to see the family doctor, he told me that he thought it was my parenting and that I was inconsistent with my parenting skills. He said that I should go to a parenting class since I was a single mom."

In situations like this, Jessica Gavin of the PANS Research and Advocacy Initiative suggests focusing on strong communication and advocacy skills. She recommends presenting your child's physical symptoms and asking their advice and thoughts. Share research on P/P and say, "I heard of this. What do you think?" Be sure to be grateful and thank them.

"This is a huge piece and so many people would get more help in their local communities if they communicated better with their doctors," Gavin said. "Doctors don't want you to tell them what it is or how to fix it. They want to help you, but they want to fix it. The trend is changing, but even when doctors believe [in P/P], they don't know what to do."

Do you remember the story of my friend who insisted on the strep test with the pediatrician who originally refused to administer it? Because of this encounter, the pediatrician's office has since done training on P/P and the doctors in the practice now have a baseline knowledge of the disease. Your insistence and education can and will make a difference when done the right way.

The longer a child has P/P and underlying illnesses, the harder it can be to eradicate it. If you spend time seeing inexperienced physicians, you may find yourself on a spinning hamster wheel and may likely end up spending more money overall for tests that were unnecessary. If you have a pediatrician who continues to dismiss your concerns, it will simply be a waste of precious time and energy to convince them otherwise. You are much better off seeking out a specialist or another P/P-friendly pediatrician. (Again, resources at the end of this book can point you in the right direction.)

In addition to P/P specialists being expensive, there can be months-long waits to see them. Make the appointment now and consider holding off on getting opinions from other physicians until after that first appointment.

While waiting three months to see an LLMD who was a P/P specialist, we decided to see an infectious disease doctor. That doctor discredited the results of the previous Lyme test and ordered another round of bloodwork, all of which came back negative. The doctor refused to acknowledge our daughter's multiple symptoms and encouraged us to see a psychiatrist. It was a waste of time and money and only left us more frustrated.

"I can't tell you how many times parents have come to me after seeing five other providers – each one has told them something different and they are so confused and don't know which path to take," said Jana Roso of Alive and Well. She supports the idea of seeing a P/P specialist instead of getting opinions from multiple providers.

Before we had the P/P diagnosis, we had also hired a therapist to observe our daughter in our home to help figure out her behavior. After only a half-hour, the therapist told us that if we could not find an underlying medical reason for the behavior, she would diagnose her with bipolar or dissociative identity disorder (previously known as multiple personality disorder).

"Unfortunately, there are some clinics claiming to be experts in the area of PANS/PANDAS, but they tell most parents that their child just needs behavioral therapy or psychiatric evaluation," said Roso.

If there is not a P/P specialist near you and you are unable to travel to one or you cannot afford a specialist, do your research online and bring lots of materials from reputable sources to the physician you do end up seeing. Call the physician first and ask about their thoughts and beliefs regarding P/P. Many parents have waited for an appointment with a particular physician, only to find out during the meeting that they don't believe in P/P and aren't open to hearing otherwise. Calling ahead of time and finding out if the doctor has treated other P/P patients or is open to learning more about the disorder will save you time and energy. Again, the more information you can bring, coupled with your notebook, the more likely you are to get an accurate diagnosis.

Lastly, try to pay it forward to future families. A mom from Texas said that while trying to get her son evaluated, they went to a neurologist who had never treated P/P, but kept an open mind about it.

"I begged him to try longer-term antibiotics, even though my son's strep infection was gone. He hesitantly agreed to it," she said. "Once starting on the antibiotics, my son didn't rage for 40 days. Before that, he was raging every few days. We ended up finding a PANDAS specialist, but I wrote the neurologist a letter thanking him for helping us because those antibiotics ended up leading to our next steps. I genuinely wanted to express our appreciation, but I also wanted to make it easier for the next family walking through his door."

Diagnosis Criteria

PANDAS is a clinical diagnosis based on six distinct criteria developed by the National Institute of Mental Health (NIMH). A "clinical diagnosis" means that there are no definitive labs or tests that can be used to diagnose PANDAS. According to the NIMH, the diagnosis criteria include:

- Presence of OCD, a tic disorder, or both
- Pediatric onset of symptoms (i.e., age 3 to puberty)
- Episodic course of symptom severity (dramatic ups and downs in the severity of the OCD and tics)

- Association with group A Beta-hemolytic strep infection (GAS), such as a positive throat culture for strep or history of scarlet fever
- Association with neurological abnormalities, such as physical hyperactivity or unusual, jerky movements that are not in the child's control
- Very abrupt onset or worsening of symptoms

PANS is also a clinical diagnosis. The working criteria for diagnosis includes the following:

- Abrupt, dramatic onset of OCD or severely restricted food intake
- Concurrent presence of additional neuropsychiatric symptoms (with similarly severe and acute onset), from at least two of the following seven categories:
  - Anxiety
  - Emotional lability and/or depression
  - Irritability, aggression, and/or severely oppositional behaviors
  - Behavioral (developmental) regression
  - Deterioration in school performance, related to ADHD-like symptoms, memory deficits and/or cognitive changes
  - Sensory or motor abnormalities

  - Somatic signs and symptoms, including sleep disturbances, enuresis or urinary frequency
- Symptoms are not better explained by a known neurologic or medical disorder, such as Sydenham's chorea, systemic lupus erythematosus, Tourette disorder or others

Important to note is that while the NIMH criteria for PANDAS diagnosis specifies pediatric onset, there is no age limit for the diagnosis for PANS. Typically, symptoms begin during a child's grade-school years; however, initial symptoms can also present during adolescence.

While there is no one conclusive test for P/P, medical providers can perform basic bloodwork, conduct viral and bacterial testing, run a Cunningham Panel™ test, and look at symptom scales. We will discuss each of these later in this chapter. However, at the end of the day, PANDAS and PANS are clinical diagnoses based on medical history, signs, symptoms and laboratory results that cannot be explained by any other medical or neurological disorders. This is where finding the right physician to diagnose your child is critical.

Finding the Underlying Cause

Once you get the diagnosis of P/P, it may take time to figure out the underlying condition, but finding the root cause is critical to treatment. The root cause may be strep, mold, Lyme, tickborne co-infections, toxins, etc. If you do not treat the root cause, P/P will not go away. It may take a few different blood tests, stool samples or urine tests. None of these are pleasant. In addition, results may take weeks.

It is also worth noting that once an illness has broken the blood-brain barrier and has inflamed the brain, the body remembers, and it may happen again. This is where new or different illnesses may cause flares in your child in the future.

Since PANDAS is caused by strep, if you suspect strep is the cause, you could start by visiting your pediatrician and requesting a rapid strep test as well as the overnight culture. Depending upon those results, you could also request bloodwork for Anti-Streptolysin O (ASO) and Anti-DNase B. Both tests help determine whether your child has had a recent strep infection. Taking both tests are very important because a child may have been recently treated with antibiotics for strep, no longer test positive on a rapid strep test or throat culture, yet still have high bloodwork titers. According to Mayo Clinic Laboratories, performing both tests is also justified because a significant portion of individuals with normal antibody titers for one test will have elevated antibody titers for the other test. Doing both tests will reduce the percentage of false negatives.

As I mentioned, strep can also occur around the anus and rectum. If you see a red rash around these areas, you will want to request a skin swab test. Perianal strep (also called perianal streptococcal dermatitis or perianal streptococcal cellulitis) is a bacterial infection of the skin around the anus and rectum, which can also spread to the vulva or penis.

If your child tests positive for strep, you will want to get everyone else in the family tested. It is possible that others in the family are carrying strep and are asymptomatic. If this is the case, your child will not get better, as she may be reinfected by other family members, unless they are also treated.

There are several lab tests you can request from your physician to help determine the underlying cause of PANS (remember, PANS is caused by illnesses other than strep). According to PANDAS Network, some of the tests that you can discuss with your physician include the following:

- Complete blood count (CBC) with differential (CBC measures white blood cells, while the differential will break out the type of white blood cells)
- Comprehensive metabolic panel
- Mycoplasma pneumonia IgG (can result in "walking pneumonia")

- IgG, IgA and IgM levels
- Coxsackie A and B titers
- Epstein Barr virus
- Herpes simplex virus (HSV)
- Influenza
- Parvovirus B19 (can result in fifth disease)
- Varicella (chickenpox)
- Yeast overgrowth
- Allergies (food and environmental)
- Mycotoxins (includes molds)
- Parasites

The Cunningham Panel™ is another test that clinicians use to help diagnose autoimmune neuropsychiatric disorders. The panel, developed by Dr. Madeleine Cunningham, an internationally recognized leader in neuropsychiatric disorders research and other infection-induced autoimmune disorders, consists of five tests. According to Moleculera Labs, which conducts the tests, the Cunningham Panel™ measures "the levels of circulating autoantibodies associated with certain neurologic and psychologic symptoms. Elevated levels indicate that symptoms may be due to an infection-driven autoimmune problem, rather than a neuropsychiatric disorder."

It is important to note that the Cunningham Panel™, while helpful for diagnosis by a physician, is not required for diagnosis. Personally, we never ordered the panel of test for either of our daughters and I have spoken with other parents who also have forgone this test. It is worth mentioning that the test costs nearly $1,000, and Moleculera currently does not participate in any insurance plans, though some may make an exception with a fight. You will need to consider whether the benefit of the test outweighs the cost for your particular situation.

Lyme Disease and Co-Infections

If you suspect that Lyme disease or other tickborne infections are a possible cause of P/P for your child, it is important to test for which ones are most likely, based on your child's symptoms.

The Centers for Disease Control and Prevention (CDC) recommends a two-part screening test for Lyme disease. The first part, ELISA, measures levels of antibodies against Lyme bacteria. According to the CDC, if the test comes back negative for the antibodies, no further test is recommended. If the ELISA is positive or unclear, a second test is recommended. However, according to the Global Lyme Alliance, the ELISA is falsely negative nearly 50% of the time, so the group highly recommends moving on to the next test.

The second test to confirm Lyme disease is the Western blot test. Like the ELISA, it also tests for antibodies;

however, it reports reactivity against a panel of 10 different proteins found on the Lyme bacteria. According to the CDC, five of the bands must be positive for an overall positive Western blot test result. The Global Lyme Alliance estimates that the blot test is approximately 80% accurate. It is also worth noting that, according to the CDC, antibodies regularly persist in the blood for months or even years after the infection is gone; therefore, these tests alone cannot be used to determine if the patient has healed.

Given that an increasing number of ticks have been found to carry and transmit multiple infections, it is important to test for co-infections as well. The tests and treatments for these co-infections are different than those for Lyme disease.

Co-infections vary in their symptoms and some are more prevalent in different areas of the country. To get the most accurate test results, I recommend working with an LLMD (Lyme Literate Medical Doctor) to test for the most likely of the following co-infections at specialty labs, such as IGeneX or Galaxy Diagnostics:

- Babesia Microti
- Babesia Ducani
- Bartonella
- Ehrlichia
- Anaplasmosis
- Borrelia Miyamotoi

- Rocky Mountain Spotted Fever

After you meet with a practitioner and get a P/P diagnosis as well as determine the underlying illnesses, be sure to tell your child about P/P in a way that makes sense to her. Your child already knows something is not right. Letting her know that there is a medical reason will help reassure her that she is on the path to treatment and you are working on finding the answers. In the Additional Resources section at the end of this book you'll find a couple of books written specifically for children to help them better understand P/P.

Chapter 3: Treatment

There are many different avenues of treatment for P/P, and treatment will vary based on the underlying condition, type of physician and the child. Treatment may also differ based on how long your child has had the illness and the strength of her immune system.

Research and explore all treatment options, including conventional medicine, homeopathy, integrative medicine, functional medicine, dietary changes, IVIG and low-dose immunotherapy. The options can be overwhelming. It will be up to you to determine which is the right fit for your child and your family. In addition, each child may respond differently to different treatments. The first treatment you try may not be the only treatment you try.

Treatment Options

Conventional medicine traditionally uses drugs, such as antibiotics, anti-virals, anti-inflammatories and steroids to treat P/P and the underlying conditions.

Another conventional treatment option a doctor might consider for your child is a tonsillectomy. Though there haven't been any published studies on P/P kids, there have been unpublished findings and anecdotal evidence to show benefits for some kids.

The use of SSRIs (Selective Serotonin Reuptake Inhibitors) might also be considered. According to the PANDAS Physicians Network, these medications should be started at a very low dose, a quarter or less of that used for a non-P/P child. Though side effects are generally well managed, caution should be exercised, and kids should be monitored closely for suicidal thoughts or behaviors.

With homeopathy, there is a belief that the body can cure itself with the use of natural substances to stimulate the healing process. The idea is that a substance that brings on symptoms in a healthy person can, in very small doses, treat an illness with similar symptoms. A homeopath will likely prescribe a remedy specific to your child.

The functional medicine approach uses a biology-based approach that focuses on identifying and addressing the root cause of the disease. This approach is based on the idea that each symptom may be one of many contributing to a person's illness.

In integrative medicine, physicians use a combination of practices and treatments, including both alternative and conventional medicine.

Low-Dose Immunotherapy (LDI) is a sort of blending of immunotherapy (think of "allergy shots") and homeopathy. LDI is designed to promote immune tolerance to various antigens/immune triggers in order to stop unnecessary and inappropriate immune reactivity, thereby decreasing symptoms. For example, there are antigens available for foods; bacteria including strep, Bartonella and Mycoplasma; viruses such as Coxsackie; and parasites like Babesia.

Intravenous Immunoglobulin (IVIG) is a therapy that can help people with weakened immune systems fight off infection. It combines immunoglobulins donated by thousands of different people to give the patient antibodies that the body is not making on its own. IVIG is given through a vein in the arm over the course of 2-4 hours. It can be done at a medical facility or at home. According to the PANDAS Physician Network, a single course of IVIG is often sufficient to produce significant improvements in symptoms. Some parents find that their child needs multiple rounds.

The first specialist we saw for my daughters strongly believed that only a combination of antibiotics could get rid of Lyme and other tickborne illnesses as well as P/P. For one of my daughters, these treatments worked well. We were able to curb the worst P/P symptoms within a few months with no negative side effects.

Many of the parents I have spoken with agree that sometimes a traditional treatment using antibiotics works, but it might take a few tries to find the right type of antibiotics, in the right combination, at the right dose level. It is really important to manage your expectations upfront that the first treatment may not be the ultimate solution.

However, for my other daughter, antibiotics caused a whole host of other side effects and issues, including a bacterial infection in the small intestine. For her we needed to switch to a more functional and integrative medicine approach.

Jessica Gavin of the PANS Research and Advocacy Initiative agrees. "What works for one doesn't always work for another," she said.

Some treatment paths may get your child to 95%, but you may still need to switch approaches at some point to get ultimate healing. Keeping an open mind and staying in the loop on what is working for others in a support group will help you make that transition easier when the time is right.

Dr. Sarah Griesemer, a licensed psychologist who provides therapy to parents of P/P kids, said that many parents she sees tend to choose one track for treatment. "They want to only use holistic health solutions and focus on supplements and diet, or they are focused on using psychiatric medication to manage behavior," she said. "The parents that seem to have the most success, in my opinion, are the ones willing to do a little of everything.

"They will involve a psychiatrist to help the child manage anxiety and depression, and the trauma of this disorder; they will adjust the child's diet and sensory diet as well as they can; they will loop in medical professionals to take an aggressive tactic with antibiotics; and they use therapy to help manage issues around OCD and self-esteem. Because this disorder affects so many aspects of the child's life and body, it requires a very wide support system."

No matter which treatment you go with, all of them have one thing in common: Healing correctly takes time. Your child has a dysregulated immune system, and it needs to be modulated. You may see slow and steady progress for a few days only to go backward the next. This is normal. Treatments do not work overnight, and progress does not happen in a straight line.

You will likely know when treatment is working based on your child's behavior and her own observations. One child with PANDAS was able to articulate the impact of medicine on his brain while he was healing. "The white pill is magic," he said. "My brain is cold. Before I started taking the white pill, my brain was burning all the time. I didn't know I could feel this well. I didn't know my brain could be cold." Keep your eyes and ears out for verbal and non-verbal expressions of your child's improvement.

The Emergency Room

There may come a time when you are desperate for help managing your child who is psychologically spiraling out of control, despite your best efforts. Some parents opt to take their child to the Emergency Room at the local hospital. This option might be necessary for safety but also comes with risks.

Many times, the physicians in the ER are not educated on P/P. Therefore, they might generate a mental illness diagnosis and encourage you to place your child in a psychiatric ward for a period of time. Or they may prescribe drugs that treat mental illness, which may help temporarily but won't get at the root illness causing P/P.

This may prompt others to call Child Protective Services (CPS) to evaluate your situation. Again, these are individuals who generally are not educated in P/P. Working with a P/P specialist and avoiding the ER, if at all possible, is preferred for these reasons. However, if your child is at risk of hurting themselves or others, it goes without saying that a visit to the ER might be unavoidable.

Treatment Costs

Most treatments are likely to be expensive, if not for the cost of the treatment itself then due to the length of time that your child needs to be on it. Remember, you may pay more in time and money bouncing around between inexperienced doctors who are unsure how to test and treat the underlying illnesses of P/P.

We consider ourselves lucky. My husband has had good-paying jobs and medical coverage. Even so, one of the conventional drugs for just one of the tickborne illnesses was nearly $500 per month. Both of my daughters were on that medicine for four months at a time and for multiple rounds. In addition, our children were on multiple prescriptions. We cut back on a lot of non-essential spending that year and canceled vacations. I am truly grateful that we could afford it. Being able to recognize things we were grateful for during this difficult time was one of our silver linings.

In the first year of uncovering and treating both my daughters for Lyme, Bartonella and Babesiosis as well as P/P, we spent approximately $15,000 on doctor visits, tests, procedures and treatments. The more you can focus on getting the right doctor who knows what to test for and has a treatment plan you are comfortable with, the less costly this journey may be.

For some children who don't respond to antibiotics, homeopathy or functional and integrative medicine treatments, you may need to explore IVIG. It can be a battle to get insurance to cover this expensive treatment. I highly recommend reaching out through Facebook groups if this is a treatment you are considering in order to get the latest costs and perspective on it, as well as tips on how to get it approved through your insurance.

Regardless of the treatment approach you choose, you should ask your physician whether to introduce medicines or supplements one at a time. If you introduce them all at once and your child has a reaction, positive or negative, you may not know which one was the cause. Therefore, your doctor may recommend introducing one supplement or medicine at a time for a few days while tracking any changes in behavior or physical condition in your symptom journal.

We did not know this at first. We put our daughter on all the medicines recommended by the doctor at once, and within a few days she felt absolutely awful. We did not know what was causing it, so we had to take her off of all of them and start over again, slowly, one at a time. We wasted time and resources (remember, those medicines are expensive!). Please learn from our mistakes. You will be excited to get started on treatment and to see results, but remember this is a marathon, not a sprint.

Supportive Measures

There are some supportive measures you can take to help assist your child's recovery, including encouraging plenty of sleep, healthy eating habits and detoxing.

Importance of Sleep

While you sleep, your body can make more white blood cells that can attack the viruses and bacteria that hinder the healing process. Your immune system relies on sleep to be able to fight harmful substances. So, setting a stricter sleep schedule can be very beneficial, despite your child's protests.

That said, P/P can cause significant sleep disturbances, as can some of the underlying conditions. One of my daughters had trouble falling asleep, while another daughter had trouble staying asleep. We didn't get much sleep for a few months! My husband and I took shifts. He would stay up late putting the younger one to bed while I would deal with the middle-of-the-night wakings. Some nights it felt like we had infants all over again.

After we would put one daughter to bed, she would come downstairs and complain that she could not sleep. After many nights of bringing her back upstairs to her bedroom only for her to reappear in the family room minutes later, we gave up. For weeks, she would put a blanket and pillow on the floor behind the couch and fall asleep. Under normal situations would this be acceptable to us? Absolutely not. However, this was not a normal situation and we recognized that it would pass and that her getting enough sleep was far more important than where that sleep took place. As my mother would say, "Pick your battles."

One of my friends had the opposite sleep issue with her daughter. She would sleep 20 hours a day if they let her. They would often wake her to keep her on a schedule. "With brain healing going on, it is hard to find a magic amount of sleep hours to help restore without overdoing it," she said. "This was critical for us."

Dietary Support

Healthy eating habits can also help promote healing. Many practitioners will suggest a diet with a reduction of sugars and inflammatory foods, like dairy and gluten. I recognize that this is not always easy to implement with a child, especially a younger one, but even a few changes can add up to a big difference.

You know your child. If explaining the rationale behind making changes will help her get on board, then definitely share the proposed changes. If not, then perhaps swapping the regular chicken nuggets for the gluten-free ones might go unnoticed. Do what you can and do not stress about what you cannot.

One of my daughters has recently been battling P/P symptoms, and our practitioner suggested a low-sugar, grain-free, dairy-free diet. As a young teen, this was far from appealing to her, but knowing it would help the bloating and discomfort she was feeling helped her consider the dietary changes. I offered to do it with her, and that made all the difference. We have found new foods to enjoy together. In fact, for a while we had "date nights" where we enjoyed a date roll covered in coconut for dessert.

Detoxing

Detoxing is a critical piece of healing as well. As your child takes medicine and it begins to work, it creates "die-off" of illness in the body. Often times, the rapid "die-off" releases more toxins than the body can clear naturally through the liver and kidneys. According to LymeDisease.org, when this happens, it is called a Jarisch-Herxheimer Reaction (JHR), or "herxing." During herxing, a patient experiences an increase in symptoms following treatment. While herxing is often tied to treatment of Lyme disease and other co-infections, some parents report herxing when treating other illnesses.

In order to minimize a herxing reaction, it is important to detox the body. Detoxing helps the vital organs cleanse themselves of the toxins and enables the liver to function appropriately in getting rid of them.

As counterintuitive as this sounds, your child's symptoms may get worse at the beginning. This is due to the die-off of toxins. By detoxing, you are able to get those toxins out of the body faster and help aid recovery and relieve the symptoms.

The most common suggestions that I have heard of and embraced are Epsom salt baths and activated charcoal. Epsom salts now come in a variety of scents and are even available in bubble bath!

Activated charcoal is available over the counter in powder and capsule form. It absorbs toxins from the body and helps excrete them. It is important to note that it can prevent your body from digesting food and absorbing nutrients. It can also make medications and supplements less effective. So, it is very important that you take it two hours before or after meals, medications or supplements. Be sure to talk with your physician about the right dose for your child.

Another detoxing option is food-grade bentonite clay, which is a natural clay with a fine, soft texture. It can be added to food or drinks or put in the bath. Bentonite clay absorbs materials in the digestive tract by sticking to their ions or molecules, and as the clay leaves the body, it takes the toxins with it. Again, talk to your physician about the right dose for your child.

Recently, Alka-Seltzer Gold® was brought to my attention as a good detoxing option. Alka-Seltzer Gold® contains sodium bicarbonate (baking soda) and potassium bicarbonate, both of which are natural alkalines that can assist with eliminating toxins. It is not recommended for children under 12, so check with your doctor before trying it. The taste may be a turn-off for some, so you may want to mix it with juice instead of water or add lemon to it. Similarly, many parents report success with a pinch of plain baking soda added to water.

If your child takes antibiotics or supplements, your doctor may also recommend taking probiotics to help replenish the good bacteria in the gut. There are many different probiotic strains, strengths and forms available. Consult with your physician about which probiotic is right for your child. Like the activated charcoal, probiotics should be taken two hours before or after antibiotics so that the antibiotics do not kill off the good bacteria that you are replenishing with the probiotic.

A core treatment prescribed for brain inflammation includes ibuprofen (e.g., Advil®, Motrin®). Ibuprofen is a non-steroidal anti-inflammatory drug (NSAID) that works by reducing hormones that cause pain and swelling in the body. In this case, it helps with brain inflammation. Because it is an NSAID, regular long-term use may cause liver and kidney damage, so be sure to discuss appropriate dosing for your child with your doctor. Some other patients find naproxen (e.g., Aleve®) to be a longer-term option. There are also some alternative, natural remedies that you can explore with an integrative or functional medicine doctor.

If your child is experiencing brain fog, one remedy that my daughter and others have found incredibly helpful is DHA. DHA is an omega-3 fatty acid that research has shown is essential for brain development and has also been linked to reduced inflammation.

My daughter was having difficulty reading for school, as the words and paragraphs were appearing smushed together. She found that taking DHA really helped reduce this issue and her brain fog. If your child is having cognitive issues, this might be a supplement that you talk to your doctor about. If your child is sensitive to fish oils, you may want to try a vegan alternative, made from algae.

Relapsing

In the opinion of Dr. Griesemer, "This disorder can get better and, yes, your child can get to a functional place. This is not a disease that is cured, unfortunately, but instead is a chronic autoimmune disorder that has changed how your child's body functions."

While you see your child improve with proper treatment, do not be surprised if you see her relapse and experience flares. This is completely normal. My daughter will have a great day or two and then completely lose it because she is overly tired or hungry, or her allergies are acting up. It seems like there are little, unexpected triggers that may set her off.

One of my daughters used to suffer episodes before coming down with a cold or with the onset of seasonal allergies. My other daughter would experience episodes when she had a loose tooth. Other P/P parents have mentioned that they see their child have episodes when there is a full moon.

The good news is that over time you will learn what flares, episodes and relapses look like, and you will be able to see them coming a mile away and be able to begin treating them before they are full blown.

Fight-or-Flight Response Regulation

Did you know that one of the best tools you have at your disposal to help your child function and feel better faster is learning to regulate your own nervous system?

Yup! Our body's state (whether we are relaxed, or activated, or in fight-or-flight mode) is directly influenced by what is happening around us; and our own body's state can affect the nervous system of other bodies nearby.

"If your child's nervous system is in a fight-flight mode, then it might trigger that mode in your own body," Dr. Griesemer explained. "Likewise, learning to turn off your fight-or-flight response in your own body can help your child's body switch out of fight-or-flight. This is a powerful tool that you have that we often overlook when we ignore the relational way that mammals' bodies function."

While this is great advice, it can be difficult to achieve in the moment, and therefore may require a bit of practice on the parents' part. It could be counting down from 10, taking three big breaths, or walking away to cool down for a few minutes. There are many different techniques to diffuse the situation, but all will require you to modify your behavior before expecting your child to change. More techniques will be covered in the chapter on self-care.

Chapter 4: Expectations

As you have probably already realized, P/P will turn life upside-down not only for your child but also for your entire family. Setting expectations for yourself, your P/P child, your other children, and your spouse or partner will help you endure the rollercoaster ride.

First and foremost, do your best to try to accept this new, unwelcomed and overwhelming reality you've found yourself in. You are doing everything you can to help your child, but in the meantime, life will be different for everyone in the household. It might last a while, but it is temporary. Make peace with it. Now is not forever.

"Most families who come to me for help are struggling with figuring out how much to expect of their PANDAS child," Dr. Griesemer said. "They have a memory of what that child used to be able to do and vacillate between thinking their child cannot do anything and needs extensive support, and thinking that their child is being manipulative and taking advantage of the situation.

"This disorder is so different from others because of the way it waxes and wanes. It's a moving target for parents to manage, where they must constantly adjust their expectations of their child day by day and week by week. Often, they need help seeing their child objectively and figuring out, 'What can my child manage right now?'"

Your child now has special needs. She will require more of your time, patience and love. Remember that your child's behavior is a result of the illness and is not who she is – she does not like the negative behavior either. She wishes she could control her behavior, but she cannot. As her parent, it is important to try to stay calm and patient. This can be especially hard in the moment. But by staying calm, you can help the situation from escalating further. Your child is likely having a harder time dealing with the situation than you are.

At the beginning of our journey, my daughter was having multiple P/P raging episodes a day. It was absolutely exhausting. Often by the time my husband got home from work, I was at my breaking point. We worked hard on our communication, and on the days when I was ready to lose it, I would let him know before he left the office so that he could immediately step in and I could take a break and recharge. Letting him know that I expected his help allowed him to be prepared to jump in on those days. We became a tag team, and it made all the difference.

A woman I used to work with had an expression: "Be a scientist, not a judge." This advice is relevant when dealing with your child. Try to approach every situation from a point of understanding. Ask questions to understand what is triggering the behavior. While you will be tempted to reason with your child, they cannot be reasoned with while having an episode. Their brain is in fight-or-flight mode, so they cannot comprehend reasoning. Wait until the child is out of an episode to discuss the behavior.

Another strategy that I used to help myself deal with my child's behavior was to treat her as though she was my client. This mental shift in thinking and perspective forced me to stay calm, patient and professional. As much as I'd like to at times, I would never yell at a client.

Dr. Griesemer encourages parents to "remember that behavior comes from a need. Because of how the brain inflammation works in kids with PANDAS, they quickly react to their needs behaviorally and are unable to verbalize their needs or delay their responses.

"Trust that when your child yells for the volume to get turned down on the car radio, it's because she cannot manage that level of stimulation on their nervous system any longer. She isn't being a brat or trying to make you miserable, as much as it might seem that way. Her brain is on fire and cannot manage as much stimulation as your body can manage or as much as she used to be able to manage. For a child with PANDAS/PANS, sometimes a little thing is more than she can manage in that moment. Trust your child is doing their best to tell you what they need through their behavior."

Now is a good time to relax the household rules to help reduce episodes. For us it meant being flexible with where our daughter fell asleep. For others it might be bedtime, how chores are managed, what the child wears and how frequently clothes are washed, or how frequently the child brushes her teeth. Remember, this is temporary. Your child will eventually sleep in their own bed and wear clean clothes daily, but right now you want to keep them as calm as possible.

Take Time to Grieve

"Parents will need time to grieve the loss of what they thought parenting would be like, and what their lives would be like," explained Dr. Griesemer. "I cannot emphasize enough the pain and waves of grief that parents of PANDAS/PANS kids experience, and how important it is to honor and make space for this grief process.

"Parents also will need help and support accepting that this is a chronic disorder. Some parents can get so fixated on 'fixing' PANDAS that it can have the unintentional side effect of making their child feel like a problem that needs to be solved. Recognize that you are all victims of PANDAS, even your PANDAS child, and that you are all grieving and suffering together. By grieving with your PANDAS child, you make the problem PANDAS and not them."

School and Extra-Curricular Activities

It is important to set expectations in terms of school and extra-curricular activities. While some P/P children are able to make it through the school day, others are not. My daughter would make it through the school day but have a meltdown the millisecond she got in the car at pickup. Some days we didn't make it out of the school parking lot. I would have to pull into a parking spot in order to calm her down just enough so that I could drive home safely.

I had to change my expectations and reframe what school pickup would look like. I had to accept that she was doing everything she could to keep it together all day inside school and seeing me at pickup was the first chance she would have to let her guard down and release. Once I accepted this new normal, I came armed with snacks and water. I moved or canceled extra-curricular activities. I accepted that after school would be for decompressing, and that was just fine.

Getting out of the house can be difficult due to the various symptoms that your child may be experiencing. It could be her inability to wear socks or shoes due to sensory issues or her OCD rituals, fixations or fears of something. It may not even be obvious to you or your child why leaving the house is so impossible. One friend told me that her son suddenly "just couldn't" leave the house, even to go out to dinner as they had hundreds of times before he got sick.

If you suspect that your child will not be able to handle an outing or a get-together, listen to your gut. These are not the first nor the last get-togethers that you will have to cancel. It's OK. Remember, this too shall pass!

When my daughter was very sick from the tickborne illnesses and PANS, we had to cancel all her extra-curricular activities. While she loved gymnastics at the time, she wasn't up for the activity. She wasn't comfortable putting on the leotard. Same with soccer. Her stomach hurt too much to run around, and she couldn't commit to the team to show up for practices or games.

While it was a tough decision, pulling her from the extra-curricular activities ended up allowing her to give her body the rest it needed to recover. She also ended up reading more and discovering her passion for writing. Remember I mentioned there would be silver linings? This was one for her.

Family and Friends

If it is not already obvious, most family, friends and co-workers are not going to understand what you are going through. They may listen and offer unsolicited advice on your parenting style to try to be helpful, but they likely cannot truly comprehend what you and your family are going through. They are not living it day to day. They do not see what goes on behind the closed doors of your home. The best you can do is educate them by sharing articles and resources.

On www.panslife.com, a website by Lisa Kilion that offers support and education to families facing P/P, there is a fabulous blog titled "Letter to Grandparents and Other Family Members." In the letter, she tackles 10 myths and realities when it comes to P/P. It is incredibly powerful and can be shared with not only grandparents and family members but also friends.

Bystanders

A big challenge can be what to say to bystanders during a flare or episode. My friend shared a memory where one time she was at the mall with her two children. Her daughter with P/P was hurting her younger sibling. She had to physically restrain her P/P child right there and then. A woman walking by accused her of abuse. She responded calmly with, "Thank you for your concern. My child is healing from a brain injury and at times needs to be restrained for her and others' safety, but I assure you she is fine." I thought this was the perfect response in the moment and one we can all embrace during those difficult moments.

Siblings

P/P will have an impact on your other children. They may have trouble understanding why their sibling is not behaving well and constantly throwing tantrums. They may feel like their sibling has completely changed. They might get hit or scratched unexpectedly. They may start to communicate that they do not understand why their sibling does not like them. It is heart-breaking to hear this sentiment of one child about another.

To help alleviate the family strain, you may want to consider family counseling with a therapist aware of P/P. We did counseling for both of our children alone, together, and as a family. My husband and I also did couples therapy. It helped us get through the rough days. Therapy can also be helpful for the P/P child to deal with anxiety, a common symptom.

A strategy to help keep your non-P/P children safe is to encourage them to play in a separate part of the home during an episode or go to a friend's or neighbor's house. This will keep the siblings safe and reduce the animosity the siblings will have toward your child with P/P.

A single P/P parent I spoke with had a solid safety plan in place. She had locks on the sibling's door and if the P/P child started showing signs of a bad episode, the sibling would go into her room with a cell phone and lock the door. If things got particularly bad, the mom could ask the sibling to call a trusted, supportive neighbor or friend for help.

"I can't take care of my PANDAS son if I'm guarding and protecting my daughter," she explained. The plan even worked when the mom was away from home.

"My daughter called me while I was at the grocery store. My son had grabbed a knife and she saw his eyes had changed. She grabbed the cat and ran into her room and locked the door. She knew the safety plan and she was able to implement it."

Another strategy that we used to help ensure both of our daughters felt loved and heard, was parent/daughter days. My husband would take one child for the day and I would take the other. The kids would make a list of all the things they wanted to do with us. We would spend special time with each of them. It gave our non-P/P daughter a chance to have our individual attention without dealing with her sibling's episodes. It gave them both a chance to feel completely and utterly loved. It also gave my husband and me a chance to take turns away from the flaring child. My children loved these special days.

Emotional Support

I found that the times I was most frustrated and upset were often the times when my children needed my love and hugs the most. If your child will let you, give hugs, even when you do not feel like it. There is power in the human touch.

When you are explaining P/P to others, it is incredibly important to not talk negatively about your child, especially in front of them. Remember, they are not in control of their actions. It is not their fault. Blame the illness, not the child.

My husband and I were looking forward to our 10-year anniversary trip. We had planned it and fantasized about it for months. It was going to be a once-in-a-lifetime trip to Costa Rica, without the kids. Needless to say, it had to be canceled. It wasn't the first. It won't be the last. When it comes to taking trips, we have learned to set low expectations, invest in trip insurance, quickly mourn these canceled vacations and move on. The trips will happen, eventually.

I am not a super religious person; however, I recognize and appreciate the power of prayer. If prayer helps you get through these rough days, pray as often as needed.

Recovery

It is important to set your expectations of the recovery process. It is a not a straight line. Your child will have good days and bad days. Your child may even have a few good months or years and then experience a relapse or flare with a new infection. If you are on the lookout and expect it, you will be able to treat more quickly each time.

One mom shared this sentiment: "My son had a flare last weekend that lasted three days. Before that he was mostly stable. We can now count the rages on one hand in 12 months' time, instead of one hand in one day."

This journey is very, very hard. Some days you may feel like a failure. Remind yourself that you are not a failure. You are doing the best you can every day and that's all that can be expected.

Chapter 5: The Child's Perspective

In order to help parents understand what their children are going through, I thought it might be helpful to get insights from P/P children on how they feel when they are experiencing an episode or flare and when they are managing their symptoms. The names of the children have been changed when requested to protect their privacy.

Are you aware when you are having an episode?

"Yes. I have a parasite and have my episodes around the full moon each month." – Cash, 9

"No, not at all." – Chace, 11

"Only a little for me." – Mae, 11

"Now I am because I know what it is. Back then I didn't. In the moment, you don't realize it because you feel really upset." – Savannah, 11

"Not really. You kinda recognize that you aren't yourself, but you don't want to admit it to yourself." – Jo, 12

"Yes. Everything makes me mad. I hate to be talked to or bothered. I explode over little things and have no control over myself. I just want to be left alone." – Keaton, 13

"I am sometimes, but not always." – Sarah, 13

"That is hard to answer. I'm aware to an extent. I know what I am doing, but in my head, I have reasoning for it. Adults might not understand. It's like an on-and-off switch. It just goes on. It doesn't slowly creep in." – Maya, 14

"Sometimes. It kind of depends on the severity of the symptoms. If I start hallucinating or feel extremely depressed, then I'm pretty aware that I'm having an episode, but most often my parents have to tell me I'm in an episode and not to trust the way I'm currently feeling. Other times, I'll have subtle symptoms, such as finding it hard to think, stuttering, trouble focusing, or bad handwriting. I myself don't tend to notice those symptoms as much, but my parents do." – Daniel, 17

Do you remember having an episode?

"Yes, but I usually don't remember how it started/what started it." – Toby, 8

"Vaguely." – Jo, 12

"Kind of. It is hard to understand what is going on and hard to stop your actions." – Delaney, 13

"Most of the time, yes, because I realize how different I act." – Sarah, 13

"All the time. I feel bad that I make everyone angry and frustrated with me. I feel like I make everything worse in our family." – Keaton, 14

"I don't always remember what happens. At least not vividly." – Maya, 14

"Sometimes I'll remember having the episode. However, if it's really intense, then I don't remember much, including everything else that's happened during that time period. It's nerve-wracking because I'll struggle with large gaps of time missing." – Daniel, 17

"My memory is usually pretty bad during an episode. I remember I was in an episode, but not everything that happens." – Ellie, 17

What does your head feel like during an episode?

"Sometimes my head hurts like something is pressing on me. My head feels like I have a lot of heavy stones on it." – Lav, 7

"It feels empty, as if I can't do anything to stop it, and my nervous system is ineffective." – Will, 10

"I have a really bad headache, and trouble focusing." – Caty, 11

"It feels like there is way too much to handle with thoughts and anxiety." – Chace, 11

"It feels fine except there's a lot of voices in my head." – Mae, 11

"I feel light-headed, and I usually get a headache." – Santino, 11

"I feel really upset and mad about the situation. You scream and cry and can't take care of things maturely. You get upset without thinking about things." – Savannah, 11

"When you are having an episode, all you want to do is yell and be mad. You want it to be your way. Even if there is a solution, you don't want to drop the subject." – Jo, 12

"Your head feels full of misunderstood information. It just feels very overflowing." – Delaney, 13

"It varies, but it hurts, and I feel dizzy. If you mean mentally, I feel as if I'm going crazy." – Sarah, 13

"It feels like it's pulsing." – Keaton, 14

"It hurts. It throbs." – Maya, 14

"At some moments it feels like a waterfall of thoughts and ideas or conversation between myself and my imagination. Other times it's almost unnervingly silent or muddled and I have trouble paying attention or remembering things." – Daniel, 17

"It feels really fuzzy like I just woke up, but it's an all-day-long feeling. So, when little things that are stressful happen, it's really intense for me." – Ellie, 17

What helps get you out of an episode?

"My mom gives me relief and I like to have a bath. It usually calms me." – Lav, 7

"When I get tired and run out of energy, or Mom suggests stuff I really, really want to do. I also try to go into my room and relax or start watching a show on TV. I also sometimes will sip some Alka-Seltzer Gold® fizzy water." – Toby, 8

"My big dog, Daisy. My cat, Juno. Big, tight bear hugs from Mom and Dad." – Caty, 11

"Just go to a different room and calm down for 10 minutes by petting my dog or watching TV." – Chace, 11

"Mommy holding me and calming me down helps. So do funny YouTube videos." – Savannah, 11

"When my mom calms me down." – Jo, 12

"There are a couple of tools I use to help me. I lean on Jesus and my family. I find a distraction to ease the anxiety; use calming tools, fidget toys and calming apps; and spend time with my dog, Abbey." – Sarah, 13

"Meds, ibuprofen, Epsom salt baths and detox." – Keaton, 14

"Getting tired and giving up." – Maya, 14

"Steroids have been a helpful way to end episodes. They are consistent every day, but they do tend to wear me out. The effects of the steroid can usually be seen the next day and it feels like waking up." – Daniel, 17

What does a tic feel like?

"I feel that I have to move my hands and fingers in lines all the time. It feels nice but looks strange to my school friends." – Lav, 7

"When my throat is clogged, it is a bit annoying. You have to clear it. It keeps coming back and you have to do it again and again. It really bugs me." – Savannah, 11

"Tics feel like your body is forcing you to do something and you can't get out of it. When you have tics, you feel a lot of adrenaline." – Delaney, 13

"I sometimes have eye tics or throat clearing. Sometimes I don't know I'm having them and when I am aware of them, I overanalyze things and become very OCD. It makes me really coo-coo! I feel like I have to suppress myself and try to be normal, and sometimes I realize I can't control it and feel defeated." – Sarah, 13

"My eyes twitch. It isn't comfortable. It makes it hard to read. I know I'm doing it. My eyes are uncomfortable, and I need some way to itch them or stop them from feeling this way. It feels like there is something wrong. I need to twitch them, so I have relief, even if the relief never really comes." – Maya, 14

"Whenever I'm dealing with OCD, it's like a constant urge to do something, growing stronger until I finally do whatever needs to be done to satisfy it. I would pick at scabs on my skin and create scars because I hated the feeling of it on my skin." – Daniel, 17

"Sometimes I don't even know it's happening, and my mom will point it out. When I realize I'm having tics, it feels like lightning kind of … it's hard to explain." – Ellie, 17

How has OCD impacted you?

"I like to tear paper in small pieces and throw it up, but I do not like when my teacher tells me to stop doing it. I do not like when she tells me to stop eating pencils and erasers." – Lav, 7

"I hate OCD. It has impacted me a lot. It feels like I'm not in charge of myself anymore." – Toby, 8

"I felt like I had to bang on my wall consistently. It hurt my hands." – Chace, 11

"It impacts me a good deal. Sometimes I will erase my stuff over and over again. I feel like I have to get it perfect. When I get OCD, I will be hyper-focused on God and the Bible and I can say sorry up to one hundred times a day because I'm overwhelmed." – Sarah, 13

"Feels like I've always got to be picking at something or I feel like I'll freak out. Makes it hard for me to focus, especially on schoolwork." – Keaton, 14

"I have had two major problems with OCD. One has been obsession over the hallucinations I see often. They take the form of shadows and while my parents tell me that they're simply hallucinations and cannot harm me, I have a hard time believing them. I want to believe my parents, but during these shadow sightings I get such strong feelings of paralyzing fear and impending doom that I just can't completely accept the fact that they are just a symptom of PANDAS. The second major problem happened quite recently where I struggled with constant thoughts of suicide for a while. I have grown better, though." – Daniel, 17

"Now that I'm on the right meds, my OCD has been good. But before, it felt like if I didn't touch the door one more time it was the end of the world. I would tell myself 'one more time' a lot." – Ellie, 17

How have your math skills been impacted?

"I like numbers and blocks, but I cannot calculate." – Lav, 7

"Math seems harder because my brain moves slower." – Cash, 9

"It was super hard to do any math. I just wouldn't answer when someone asked me a question because I couldn't figure it out. I feel like I forget everything about math when I'm in a flare. When I'm feeling good, I love math. It's my favorite subject." – Toby, 9

"I couldn't do math during a flare. Simple addition and subtraction were nearly impossible, and I would have to count on my fingers. It would take forever to answer questions." – Caty, 11

"I've always been really good at math, but it's too complicated to do math when I'm sick." – Chace, 11

"My math was impacted because I wasn't able to attend school regularly. I have a hard time remembering the steps and procedures because of my lapses in attending school." – Delaney, 13

"Math is not exactly one of my strongest suits, but it's not my worst either. When I have flares, I can't exactly remember the steps of an equation and it will often take me a couple of minutes extra to finish one relatively easy problem. If I had a flare-up while learning new math concepts, I then have issues forming memories of those math concepts." – Daniel, 17

How has your reading or writing been impacted?

"I do not like to write. It makes me feel nervous. I do not like to read. I cannot concentrate on written material." – Lav, 7

"I couldn't read a book. I couldn't write. It hurt my head. It was just a bunch of letters/words I didn't even know that didn't make sense. It was a lot for my brain to handle." – Toby, 8

"I have trouble writing and reading fast." – Cash, 9

"When I'm in class and I'm writing, I will erase all the words and letters multiple times until it is perfect. I still write normal speed, but it's annoying to keep having to erase over and over again."– Savannah, 11

"I have a problem with things fitting between the lines and being perfect. My handwriting when I'm in a flare appears sloppy and uncontrollable for me. Then the OCD kicks in and I erase and often get off task because of this." – Sarah, 13

"I can't write well enough for it to be readable. My grandma, who helps me with school every day, has to take all my notes. I stutter and start and stop with reading, and have difficulty focusing on what I'm reading." – Keaton, 14

"I'll be reading, and it feels like there are a lot of words. It feels overwhelming. I'll skip a paragraph or a section, so I can start fresh. Sometimes it feels like the words are mushing together, which makes it harder to read." – Maya, 14

"When I go through a flare, I have issues with putting thoughts into words and finding a way to phrase them into complete sentences. I already have somewhat jagged handwriting, but during a flare my handwriting grows sloppier. While reading during a flare I have a harder time processing the information I'm given. I'll also have issues with remembering important tidbits that I'd read only moments ago." – Daniel, 17

"My writing is OK, I think, but when I read, I have to re-read a lot because I feel like I can't process what I've read." – Ellie, 17

Do you experience any issues with going to school?

"School was too much to handle. I wanted to be home instead. The other kids were too loud. There was too much commotion. I'm still doing virtual/homeschool. It's still hard to focus on schoolwork at home." – Toby, 8

"Since PANDAS, I hate school. It makes me more nervous. Tests make me so much more nervous than ever before. Pretty much any place other than home makes me nervous now – unless it has people that I really know and trust inside of it. Also being around other humans that I don't know really well makes me much more uncomfortable than ever before." – Will, 10

"Yes. My mom used to try to take me to school. I had a really hard time getting into the school, and would most times sit in the nurse's office. I would tic really bad. They usually had to call my mom to pick me up. Then, I tried remote learning and it was harder. I couldn't do any homework." – Caty, 11

"Yes. I feel like I can't get out of bed or out of the house. I try so hard, but just can't do it. I'd rather be at school, but the school day feels so long." – Chace, 11

"Yes. I struggle getting up and paying attention." – Santino, 11

"Even though I love school, some days I would just feel like I didn't want to go and couldn't really explain why. I had severe separation anxiety from my mom, so eventually we just started doing online school. Not only did it help with my separation anxiety and to be more confident in my grades, it was more tailored to me than public school. Also, the people there are way nicer than they were at my old school." – Sarah, 13

"Sometimes getting ready to go to school was hard because it's hard for me to wake up and I had a hard time picking out clothes that didn't bug me." – Savannah, 14

"I haven't been able to go to school for 1½ years. I miss my friends horribly. I feel so alone. In the beginning, the school fixed my schedule so I could just go part days, but I couldn't handle all the chaos in the classroom, and I'd explode and have to call home. My anxiety made me very homesick. I also had to quit football because I couldn't handle being at practice so long – my anxiety made me just want to be home. And I had been so excited to start football." – Keaton, 14

"I never had any issues going to school but during flares, schoolwork (even answering simple questions after reading literature) was challenging. I would find it hard to process information and focus during the studying.

Combined with the fact that I had a hard time understanding the questions, forming actual answers to the questions, and remembering the answers during the homework did not improve my situation. My grades would suffer, and I would get upset with myself for my failures and for having PANDAS." – Daniel, 17

"School has been a very big struggle. I haven't been to school in a year. I've tried to go back twice, but it's been too stressful. Even thinking about it sometimes is very stressful." – Ellie, 17

Do you experience any sleep issues?

"I think about scary things and it's hard to go to sleep. It takes 30 to 40 minutes. It's hard to wake up in the morning, and when I wake up, the lights feel really bright." – Cash, 9

"Sleep is much worse. I have a lot of pain through my whole body, and it makes sleeping much harder. My mind also races sometimes at night. If my parents will let me sleep in, I will sleep until afternoon because I sometimes do not fall asleep until well after midnight." – Will, 10

"I have a lot more anxiety and energy at night, so it makes it hard to fall asleep." – Chace, 11

"It used to take me hours to fall asleep." – Mae, 11

"I had some sleep issues and I had to sleep in my mom's bedroom for years. Now I'm luckily able to sleep in my own bedroom and feel safe." – Sarah, 13

"I used to have nightmares, but my treatment has helped that." – Keaton, 14

"Sometimes during flares, I will have problems with falling asleep, even when I'm exhausted. Other times I will have hallucinations of a certain shadow that causes paralysis. I struggle with accepting that the shadows are just figments of my imagination because the shadow always 'kills' me in the nightmare. I can feel my life fading and the overwhelming sense of despair and horror, yet I can never fight back due to the paralysis. Sure, I will wake up perfectly safe and alive once the ordeal is over, but the event is traumatic and indescribable." Daniel, 17

"I've had sleep issues for years. Meds have helped. Sometimes I can't fall asleep. Sometimes I can fall asleep fine but can't stay asleep or sometimes I wake up very early or sleep very late." – Ellie, 17

What advice do you have for siblings of children with PANDAS/PANS?

"Try to not make your PANDAS sibling angry or annoyed. Their reaction will be way worse than it's ever been before." – Will, 10

"Be patient. It's not their fault they are yelling at you. Sometimes you won't even do anything wrong, and they will yell. They just can't help it. It will hurt your feelings, but they still love you. Try to help them be comfortable." – Caty, 11

"Be very patient. Don't try to bug them too much. They get real sensitive about things. Don't make fun of them ever. They can't help it." – Sarah, 13

"I would tell siblings of PANDAS to remember that whatever they're seeing in their sibling during a flare or episode is not completely them. Siblings of PANDAS children should treat their sibling with patience and understanding. Their PANDAS sibling is suffering from an illness that does not define them, and the sibling is in need of encouragement and kindness. I want my siblings to know that despite whatever I say or do during a flare or episode, I still love them." – Daniel, 17

As a sibling of a PANDAS/PANS child, what advice do you have?

"It's very annoying sometimes. They like to take control over everything a lot. They always want to get their way. It helps to know each day is a different day. Maybe today my sister won't yell at me. Some alone time away from her helps too. You just do something away from them to do something you like." – Susie, 7

"Sometimes it's hard, but you have to remember it won't be forever." – Avery, 8

"Try not to be upset, but it's hard to always hear fighting and always be late for school when my brother won't get up." – Jaxsyn, 9

"Don't get in the middle. Go hide in your room or closet until the noise stops or go on a walk or on the swings." – Jo, 11

"Walk away and let your sibling calm down." – Derek, 14

Chapter 6: Support

By now you are probably well aware of how difficult the journey can be while caring for a child with P/P. It can be emotionally, physically and financially draining. It is for these reasons it is incredibly important that you have people to turn to for support.

Spouse/Partner Support

I have heard many stories where parents have divorced after breaking under the strain of P/P. It is understandable. This is probably one of the most stressful experiences you will ever encounter as a couple. At the beginning, it is possible that you and your spouse will be in different places on your perception of P/P. You may have different parenting styles that may be in conflict as well. It is incredibly important to try to get on the same page early on.

Researching P/P and sharing information may help both parents come to the same understanding about the disease. My husband and I found it most helpful to talk to another couple who had a P/P child. Giving my husband a forum to ask questions and get answers from others and not just the Internet or me was incredibly advantageous.

A good way to keep us both engaged and involved in treatment was for both of us to attend doctor's appointments, whenever possible. My husband and I think differently, so he asked the doctor questions that I never would have thought of.

"It's certainly a journey and with conflicting advice and information, it's hard to stay aligned," my husband said. "Debating is normal, but ultimately, we need to agree on how to handle the day-to-day and what treatments to seek."

Due to the emotional toll that P/P can have on a relationship, you may want to consider couples counseling. It can help facilitate your communication and help you express your feelings about the disease and its impact on your life and your family's lives. Some people don't like to talk about their feelings, but bottling them up is not beneficial. Enlisting the help of a licensed therapist can help bring out those feelings to avoid having them be the source of an argument or resentment later.

The key is to ensure you and your spouse are set up for success by addressing any issues or disagreements early on, before they create another source of tension and frustration besides P/P itself.

I look at my husband as my partner in crime in fighting P/P. We are a team. While I take on the majority of care due to my more flexible profession, I quickly and openly share when I need help and ask him to step in to give me the break I need, when I need it. This tag-team approach has helped us from getting burned out.

I'd be lying if I said we didn't fight. This is stressful. However, we try to apologize when we're wrong and remember that we are on the same team. We need to save our energy to fight P/P, not each other.

The other day my husband was up until 4 a.m. He couldn't sleep, as he was overwhelmed by how ill our daughter had been and the impacts it was having on our family relationship, my mental health and his job performance. He was getting depressed and having difficulty motivating. We talked through it for a while. I gave him permission to focus on his job and not worry about my mental state. I promised that I would let him know when I needed him and shared that I was in a good place to handle the current demands. I encouraged him to find a coffee shop and work out of the house for a day and future days, if needed, to be able to work uninterrupted.

"In our case, and for many, the P/P child will only respond to Mom, not Dad," said my husband. "This makes life harder on moms but also adds stress, guilt and helplessness for dads. While I'd love to be helpful, at times

I'm not able." It's important for partners to understand this perspective.

Sometimes, just taking a few minutes to talk about your feelings and give each other permission to take a break is enough to keep the other person going. The roles may reverse at some point in the future.

Social Media

When we first encountered P/P, there were very few resources out there. Luckily, due to the rise of social media, finding support is easier than ever. A quick search on Facebook will reveal national as well as local P/P groups. By joining a few of these groups, you will be in touch with other parents who are further along in the journey and can share their experiences, as well as other newbie P/P parents who can commiserate with your current state.

These groups are helpful to identify P/P-friendly physicians near you, or physicians who treat remotely. They can also help you identify root causes to test for and suggest supplements to explore to help with your child's particular symptoms. There is a tremendous amount of wisdom and knowledge among those who have been on this journey for a while. Reach out to them. Lean on them. Learn from them. We are here for each other.

However, I must warn you that Facebook groups do come with their own set of challenges. "Most of these

PANDAS/PANS families are getting a lot of information from the Facebook boards," said Jessica Gavin of the PANS Research and Advocacy Initiative. "It's a lifeline, but it can be conflicting and so overwhelming. But you can learn so much if you can weed through and understand the whole picture."

A mom described the experience of finding a P/P Facebook group for the first time. "I typed in PANDAS in Facebook and found a group," she said. "I was trying to make heads and tails of it. I started to read all these posts. It terrified the living daylights out of me. I felt like I had gone through hazing and orientation into a group that I didn't want to join."

However, she admits, "Support groups on Facebook have been my lifesaver. In my state, there are 30-40 families with active diagnoses right now. Finding your local support page helps you with local suggestions from psychologists to dentists. They can give you the dos and don'ts. I wouldn't have been able to find a new PANDAS specialist without it. I finally found my tribe."

Friends of Friends

With an estimated 1 in 200 children having P/P, you may know a friend who knows a friend who has a child with this illness. The more you share information and educate others on it, the more likely you may be put in touch with someone locally who is going through it.

Many families, including mine, had a very difficult time explaining P/P to other family members. According to Dr. Griesemer, "Most people in your life will not understand what you are experiencing. They will not get it when you say your child has rages. You will need to remember that you are in the middle of a battlefield and need support and backup. Because most people won't understand your life, your new job is to get really good at describing it, and to ask for help regularly."

I found the best way to educate others was to share reliable, reputable website links of information, as well as documentaries and YouTube videos. There are some great resources out there, which I list in Chapter 9. By allowing these reputable resources to be the source of education, it is more likely that others will believe the information you are sharing. At the end of the day, some family members and friends may still not believe in P/P. Don't lose hope. The friendships you gain from others on the journey will fill the gap left from those not willing to accept your child's medical condition.

There are many children with other invisible or rare health conditions, and I found that parents of those children are also a great support system. They understand the disbelief of others. They understand the struggle to educate others. They understand the difficulty of what you are going through and may be a good sounding board.

Academic Support

Navigating the educational system with a child with P/P can also be challenging, but it is important to request accommodations for your child. In order to obtain proper support at school, you should explore getting a 504 Plan or Individualized Education Program (IEP). Both can offer formal help for K-12 students. There are some differences between a 504 Plan and an IEP, and the needs of your child may impact which program will be best. In the resources section of this handbook, you will see some websites that can help you navigate obtaining in-school support.

The one thing that I found most helpful was building a strong relationship with my daughters' teachers. At the beginning of the year, I would set up conferences to talk with them about P/P. I shared information from PANDAS Network and talked to them about my daughters' specific symptoms. I asked for their help and partnership. I encouraged them to reach out to let me know if any major illnesses were going around the classroom so that I could be on the lookout for a flare or episode. I also made sure to check in periodically to see how each daughter was doing. I wanted to ensure that what the teacher was seeing at school was similar to what I was seeing at home, which was not always the case.

An unexpected support system can be the school nurse. Meeting with and educating the nurse on P/P is also very helpful. The nurse will have a pulse on what illnesses are going around the school. Providing a written request for assistance can also be very effective. My friend wrote a letter that the nurse could send out to parents in her P/P child's grade, which stated that someone in the grade has extreme reactions to illnesses, including strep, and strongly requested they keep their child home in the event of any symptoms. The nurse did send it out, and the parent and P/P child were then top-of-mind for the nurse.

If your child is anything like mine, she may end up in the nurse's office on more than one occasion. The nurse helped keep my child calm until I could come pick up on the days when she wasn't able to return to class. You may also want to inform the nurse that you are happy to speak with any other parents of children who have P/P.

Some parents find that their child is unwilling or unable to attend school for a period of time, whether it be days, weeks or months. This is normal for P/P, and you should not feel as though you are failing your child if you have to pull her from the traditional brick-and-mortar educational system in favor of an alternative method, like homeschooling, online school, tutoring or unschooling.

When my daughter was very ill, she accumulated three weeks of missed school days in just a couple of months. It was rough not only on her but also on my husband and me, who had to play rock-paper-scissors to see who was going to work from home and take care of her.

When the pandemic began, I pulled both of my daughters out of their local middle school in favor of an online school. I considered them both to be immune-compromised and I was concerned about their higher risk level for contraction as well as the long-term implications of them catching COVID-19. I was also worried that they would not be able to adapt to potential ongoing changes in the school schedule from online, offline and hybrid. Enrolling them in online school turned out to be a blessing in disguise. It provided a consistent, flexible and predictable schedule for the year.

Some online schools, like ours, might offer fewer online lessons, an ability to work at one's own pace, and to make up classes by watching videos. If my daughter doesn't feel well, she can skip the live online class and watch the video recording instead. And if she is confused, the teachers are incredibly accessible with virtual office hours and readily available text messaging.

Instead of choosing a virtual school, a friend of mine chose to hire tutors for her son. He had missed a lot of school the previous year and was a bit behind. Knowing that he was at an age when he was less likely to listen to his mom for education, she hired two tutors to rotate throughout the week for a few hours a day. Having one-on-one attention for him was perfect. It allowed him to get help on his weaknesses and get up to grade level.

At the end of the day, you need to find the right academic support based on where your child is right now. If they can manage in-person, great. If not, explore other options – there are lots out there. And remember, your child is suffering from an illness. It is OK to take time off and go slow. Your child will be fine. She will catch up when she is feeling better.

Another method to help your child survive education under the weight of P/P is unschooling. This informal learning option allows the child to choose their activities and areas of focus based on their interests. There is no formal curriculum or grades. It is likely the most flexible and self-paced educational option available.

Daycare

Many parents, single or married, do not have the ability to stay home with their P/P child. Sometimes finding daycare for these children can be difficult given the challenges that their illness can present. One way to find the best daycare for your child is to contact your state's department of health and human services and ask for a list of daycares in your community that accommodate special needs children. You can contact the state government agency responsible for childcare licensing and speak to them to gather recommendations for a daycare that will be the right fit for your child.

Medical Leave

In the event that your child needs more support and is unable to attend school or daycare due to P/P, you might want to explore whether you are eligible to take advantage of the Family and Medical Leave Act (FMLA). According to the U.S. Department of Labor, "the FMLA entitles eligible employees of covered employers to take unpaid, job-protected leave for specified family and medical reasons with continuation of group health insurance coverage under the same terms and conditions as if the employee had not taken leave."

Eligible employees are entitled to 12 workweeks of leave during a 12-month period to care of a child with a serious health condition. While this is unpaid, it might be the time you need to help get your child's health under control without losing your job.

Professional Counseling

While your child is getting medical support, she may also need emotional support during this difficult time, and it can come in a few different forms. Some children are open to speaking to a therapist, which can help them express their feelings about what they are going through. I do caution you to find a therapist aware of and supportive of a P/P diagnosis. Be sure to call prior to making an appointment to learn about their understanding of and experience treating P/P patients.

"During flares, supportive play therapy and supportive talk psychotherapy can be incredibly helpful for kids and adolescents respectively," confirmed Dr. Griesemer. "Their self-image and self-esteem are hugely impacted by this disorder, and having a person who can help them remember who they are and help them differentiate from the disorder is very important."

Some children may resist therapy while very ill with P/P, but getting therapy after medical improvement can still be beneficial. "Therapy also provides them a place that they can help process how their disorder has affected their relationships with others. When flares die down a bit, many kids need help overcoming learned behaviors that resulted from their flare or help with OCD compulsions and obsessions," said Dr. Griesemer.

In addition to play therapy and psychotherapy, your child may also benefit from sensory or vision therapy. Many P/P children have sensory issues and some therapy can help desensitize them. There are different types of therapy for sensory processing issues, including sensory integration therapy (SI), occupational therapy and sensory diet.

As for vision, my daughter experienced the crowding of words and sentences while trying to read. It would take her up to three times as long to read as another child her age. In addition, her comprehension declined. With vision testing, we were able to uncover these specific issues and implement vision therapy to reverse them.

Your child may also find it helpful to talk to another child going through P/P. A few years ago, a friend of a friend connected me to a family who was just starting out on the P/P journey. It turned out that our kids were the same age. After gaining trust with her and her child, we were able to arrange a playdate with our kids. While the kids didn't talk much about P/P, they were grateful to be in the presence of someone who knew exactly what they were going through – someone to make them feel that they are not alone.

Siblings

When dealing with P/P, it seems that nearly 100% of the family focus is on the unwell child. It's understandable. You are trying desperately to put out fires all day long with this one child. As a result, siblings can often feel angry, frustrated and neglected. Making sure we take time to acknowledge siblings and their feelings is essential.

P/P can be brutal on siblings, especially younger children who can't quite understand what is going on and why their sister or brother is suddenly acting mean, or downright cruel, toward them. Siblings need special attention and love to get through this difficult period.

When one of my daughters was going through P/P, my other daughter and I would write in a journal that we passed back and forth. It was a way to connect with her in a peaceful setting. It gave her an outlet to share her thoughts and frustrations. By writing these feelings out on paper, she was able to get them out of her head and her heart.

Another way to help reduce sibling rivalry and give attention to the sibling is to set up special one-on-one time with each parent. As you recall, we would encourage the child to pick special things that they wanted to do with one parent and then we'd do it for the day. That break from the difficult P/P world was not only helpful for the sibling but also for the parent. A day of normalcy can do wonders!

A P/P parent shared additional suggestions on managing siblings. "My advice for parents is to have age-appropriate conversations with the sibling to let them know that their brother/sister is having a hard time and to be particularly mindful of trying to give them space (physical and emotional), patience and grace. Walk away from arguments or physical altercations and tell an adult if their sibling seems out of control or overly upset at any time."

Supportive Friends

The last bit of advice is to find your people, those who will accept you at your worst. These are the friends and family who don't judge what you are going through. They are the ones who call to check in on you and might swing by with a glass of wine on a truly bad day. Lean on those friends and family. They will help get you through. Don't worry, you'll pay it forward many times over.

Additional Support

There are many ways to get the assistance you need. The most important thing, according to Dr. Griesemer, is, "Ask for help. Ask for help. Ask for help!"

Additional ideas that Dr. Griesemer shared included asking a friend to make you a meal or set up a meal train, asking a family member or close friend (who gets it!) to babysit overnight or on a weekend, or asking your boss if you can get more flexibility at work. Figure out what you need and just ask for help.

Chapter 7: Self-Care

As selfish as it may sound and feel, you can't help others until you help yourself. There is a reason why the airlines tell you to put on your own oxygen mask first before assisting your child. You'll run out of breath otherwise. The same is true when coping with P/P.

To be clear, self-care is self-preservation. It is not self-indulgence. Taking care of yourself involves taking care of both your emotional and physical state. This can look different for each and every one of us. Try to identify what you need to feel recharged.

Exercise

While exercising when you aren't in the mood can be tough, it is one of the best things you can do to improve your state of mind. When you exercise, your body releases endorphins, which are considered to be natural painkillers because they activate the receptors in the brain that help minimize discomfort. They can help bring about feelings of well-being and euphoria. In a nutshell, endorphins make people happy!

While some people go to the gym to exercise, that can be challenging due to the amount of time needed to travel there and back, as well as actually work out. Personally, I found it more helpful to use a piece of exercise equipment in the home or go for a walk or run outside. It was easier to squeeze in a quick workout, and if my child truly needed me, I was still present.

It doesn't matter what type of exercise you do, it's the fact that you do it that matters. Go for a walk, jog, bike ride or run. Go alone and listen to music that uplifts your spirit or go with a friend to escape your day. Now that my kids are older and able to stay home alone, my husband and I try to go for a walk after dinner with the dog. It not only lets us get in some exercise, but it also allows us to touch base on our day. It's like a daily mini-date.

Involving your children in the exercise can be beneficial for the whole family if your child is feeling up for it. Sometimes we'll hop on our bikes and take a ride to the local coffee shop where we'll reward ourselves with a beverage. Other times, the girls will join me to walk the dog after finishing schoolwork.

Sometimes it's hard to get started. I find if I schedule it on my phone calendar and add a few reminders, I'm more likely to stick with it. Share your desire to exercise with others. If you say it, you're more likely to do it. Another strategy is to find an exercise buddy so you can motivate each other. It can even be a friend in another state who you talk to on the phone while you walk.

When we were both struggling, my husband and I created a weekly workout challenge where we had to do cardio for five days and weight activities for four days. We agreed that we both had to complete the activities for the week to get a reward, which was an adults-only dinner or special drinks either out at a restaurant or in the backyard. By doing it together, we were able to support and encourage each other to take time off to focus on ourselves.

Sleep

Getting a good night's rest is so important for a number of reasons. According to the SleepFoundation.org, sleep appears to be critical to both physical and mental development.

"In adults, a lack of sleep has been associated with a wide range of negative health consequences, including cardiovascular problems, a weakened immune system, higher risk of obesity and type II diabetes, impaired thinking and memory, and mental health problems like depression and anxiety," according to the website.

While our P/P children often have sleep disturbances that can affect our sleep, getting a good night's sleep is critical to dealing with this illness day in and day out. There were times my husband and I would split up the night, taking turns as to who would take care of the children should they need us. Other times, my husband would be on duty for the night, so that I could go to bed early. I also embraced the weekend afternoon nap when things were quiet.

It is also very common for P/P children to want to sleep with their mother. This is related to the separation anxiety symptom. One P/P parent shared that her husband spent many nights on the couch because of it. This may temporarily impact your relationship with your partner; however, focusing on teamwork and communication will help you both get through this stage.

If you are single or your partner or spouse is not able to assist, try to have family or friends help out for a few hours every once in a while, so that you can catch up on your sleep. It will reinvigorate you and help you to better cope.

Restorative Activities

Finding activities to calm your mind and body is also beneficial to relieving stress. This could be writing in a journal, meditating, or doing yoga. It could be enjoying a hot cup of coffee and reading a good book in the morning when the house is quiet, or sipping a glass of wine and watching a good TV show after everyone else has gone to bed. Frankly, some days it could be five minutes alone in the bathroom! Having alone time to process your feelings and thoughts is critical.

One activity that I find helpful to me, as well as my children, is nightly restorative yoga and meditation. We grab our makeshift yoga gear (pillows and blankets) and do a 10-minute yoga session on an app. It has been wonderful helping my kids calm down before bed and it simultaneously gives me 10 minutes to rest and restore. You can also explore a variety of kid-friendly restorative yoga videos on YouTube to find ones that will work best for your child's age and attention span.

After yoga, each of my daughters gets into bed and listens to sleep meditation for 10 to 15 minutes. At first, they thought it was stupid. Now they love it. It really does help them relax and fall asleep (along with some melatonin or CBD). Helping them fall asleep faster allows me to get to bed earlier.

Rediscover Hobbies

It is not uncommon for the hobbies of P/P parents to fall by the wayside as they spend all of their time and energy caring for their children. However, taking time to enjoy a hobby is a great source of self-care.

I used to enjoy cooking and baking new recipes. For a while, it seemed like just another challenge or chore. But, with a change in perspective, I revisited the hobby and began trying out new recipes again. It actually felt great to get back in the kitchen enjoying what I loved. I also found such pleasure out of baking and giving away treats to others.

One of my daughters has begun joining me in the kitchen, which I love. She has become quite the chef and baker and finds the activity a good distraction. She also feels a strong sense of accomplishment afterward. This has been a silver lining for both of us.

Self-Forgiveness

As P/P takes over your life and the lives of everyone in your household, be gentle with yourself. Often, we blame ourselves for the struggles of our children. We feel guilty that we didn't protect them enough, didn't catch the illness quickly enough, haven't found the right physician, or maybe that we didn't believe that our child was really sick. Maybe you've even blamed your own genes, wondering whether you have passed along some sort of faulty immune system onto your child.

STOP. Just STOP. You are not to blame.

You are a parent of an ill child doing the best that you can. It's time to forgive yourself and let go.

Professional Therapy

In the previous chapter, we discussed the benefits of therapy and counseling for the P/P child. If you are struggling to deal with the stress of managing this illness, you may want to consider getting help from a licensed therapist to work through your own emotions. There is no shame in admitting you need help. We all do sometimes.

"Raising a child with PANDAS is complicated, exhausting and traumatic," said Dr. Griesemer. "Most of the parents I work with have a trauma response to their child, whether it's a feeling of fight-flight when their child uses a certain tone of voice, or has a certain look on their face, or starts to push their buttons. Most parents of kids with PANDAS would benefit from doing their own therapy to help them learn how to regulate their nervous system and heal from the trauma they've experienced in their own homes."

Specifically, Dr. Griesemer recommends Trauma Focused Cognitive Behavioral Therapy (TFCBT) or Eye Movement Desensitization and Reprocessing (EMDR) if it is a parent's first experience with relational trauma.

For parents who may have had previous relational trauma, such as emotional or verbal abuse during childhood or in a romantic relationship, Dr. Griesemer suggests they work with a therapist who will also help them heal from their past experience, which might be affecting their ability to handle their current situation.

There is a lot of fear and terror, often very intense, that comes with parenting children with P/P, which therapy can also address.

"Parents also struggle with how to manage the rage and physical violence exhibited by kids with PANDAS/PANS," said Dr. Griesemer. "They fear that their child will be taken away from them by Child Protective Services because of the sounds neighbors might hear and misinterpret. They fear that the child will tell a teacher that their parent restrained her, and the teacher won't understand. They fear that they will have to call 911 for help and that the police will hurt or traumatize their child. They fear their child may hurt them or a sibling. Parents often need help figuring out what a safety plan looks like and how to talk to the systems involved (i.e., school, neighbors) in their lives."

Therapy can help parents work through these fears, and this book can help you develop action plans to address these potential issues.

Relationship Building

Marriage and partnerships are hard and with parenting a P/P child it is even harder. Take time to work on your relationship. Try to spend a few minutes alone together every day to reconnect and provide each other with love and encouragement. I know finding the time isn't easy. Make it a priority. Strengthening your communication will help you both stay sane while you parent more in sync and face this illness together.

"It's very easy to focus on your PANDAS kid to the exclusion of everything else," said Dr. Griesemer. "I've seen so many marriages suffer or fall apart because of the havoc this disorder brings into a family. You must have solid adult relationships around you to support you and be your foundation in surviving this disorder.

"To do this, you must value these relationships and put time and energy into them, even when you feel that you should be focusing on your PANDAS child. I imagine that it's like being in a house where there's a room on fire, but the foundation of the house is about to crack and break. You can focus on putting out the fire in the room, but if your foundation cracks out from under you, it doesn't matter if the fire is out or not. It's a dance of giving both attention (and maybe calling in for help!) so that you're safe."

For women, having relationships with girlfriends provides them with an outlet to share problems, thoughts, feelings and successes. These relationships boost emotional and mental strength. If you're a mom, try to spend time with friends who fill your bucket. It could be a phone call when you are alone in the car or while you are walking the dog. During COVID, I've had virtual drinks via video conference with my college friends. It has given me something to look forward to during the week. A half-hour chat will do wonders for your mood.

Just Say "No"

Now is a good time to learn to say "no" to events that no longer suit you and people who don't support you. It is hard to commit to going to an event when you aren't sure whether you will be able to leave the house given your child's separation anxiety or if you will need to be home to calm your child in the event of an epic rage (which you and you alone can diffuse).

Do your best to set expectations with others. Explain what you are going through and that you will try to attend but can't guarantee you'll make it. Through this process you will learn which of your friends have empathy, patience and understanding. True friends will get it and not hold it against you.

In my experience explaining P/P to others, I have had people ask me when my daughter's treatment will be over, and when she will be better. How I wish I could have given them a timeframe, but instead I used it as an opportunity to explain how complex a disease P/P is and that it can be recurring.

Gratitude

There is a saying about raising children that the days are long and the years are short. This is even more true as a parent of a P/P child. Some days linger on endlessly with a string of P/P episodes and only a few breaks between them. On these, your darkest days, try to find something to be grateful for. Maybe it is going to the bathroom by yourself or the break you get when your child is sleeping. Maybe you are grateful for your spouse jumping in and helping out, or your other child behaving well in the face of these challenges. There is always something to be grateful for. Hold on to these thoughts. They will get you through.

As for the good days, celebrate them. It may be a day where you only had two episodes instead of four, or a day when your child kept her clothes on (yes, I am serious!). Whatever it is – celebrate it.

The past two days were amazing in our house. We had the usual sibling rivalry, but no major meltdowns. No irrational fears, anxiety or OCD. It was incredible. We were kind of on edge just waiting for the ball to drop. And it did.

On the second night, my daughter was filled with anxiety, aches and pains in new body parts, which she claimed were bothering her for weeks, and lots of yawns despite protests of not being tired. It took extra melatonin, CBD oil, numerous sleep meditations and lots of patting her back to calm her enough for her to fall asleep just after midnight. I fell asleep on her floor wrapped in a blanket. I crawled back to my own bed around 2 a.m.

It was awful. But I am still grateful to have had a couple of days of respite and hold tight to the memory and knowledge that it will happen again, hopefully more frequently.

Dr. Griesemer also recommends doing your best to celebrate the joys and victories as much as you are looking for improvement. "This disorder is like riding a wave where there will always be highs and lows, but if we spend all our time worried about the next low, we can never enjoy the high," she said.

Post-Traumatic Stress Disorder/Acute Stress Disorder

Given all the traumatic events and experiences we witness with our P/P child, it is normal to experience Acute Stress Disorder or Post-Traumatic Stress Disorder (PTSD). According to the National Center for PTSD, Acute Stress Disorder refers to the initial traumatic symptoms that arise immediately after a traumatic event, while PTSD refers to the long-term aftermath of trauma. PTSD can only be diagnosed if symptoms have lasted longer than a month.

PTSD is a mental health condition that's triggered by a terrifying event — either experiencing it or witnessing it. Symptoms may include flashbacks, nightmares and severe anxiety, as well as uncontrollable thoughts about the event.

PTSD is very real and can keep you from moving on after your child begins to heal. In fact, we can block our child's progress by holding on to our own trauma.

Dr. Griesemer agrees. "All of the parents I have worked with have described a trauma response to their PANDAS child. Most meet the criteria for Acute Stress Disorder, and some meet the criteria of PTSD."

One parent recalled, "In the middle of a PANDAS rage, my son can trigger my PTSD and I have to fight not to disassociate myself from the situation. I don't talk about it a lot. It's really difficult."

Dr. Griesemer urges all parents to reach out to a therapist who has experience working with parents whose children have P/P or autism (because of the similarity in rages).

"Most parents would benefit from sessions with a therapist to understand how their own body is being impacted by their child's behavior so they can make a decision about whether they would benefit from ongoing therapy or not," she said. "Parents should get an evaluation and learn about how to regulate their own nervous system in the face of their child's disruptive behavior."

If you feel that you may have PTSD or Acute Stress Disorder, be sure to reach out to a therapist for help. With good self-care you can begin to heal.

Chapter 8: Tips & Tricks

Managing a child with P/P is so very hard, but having a few tricks up your sleeve can be helpful. This chapter will outline a few tips to help you and your P/P child make it through each day with a few less disruptions.

Anxiety

When your child becomes anxious, the first thing that you can do is to stay calm. It might sound basic, but it's true. If you get worked up along with your child, things will likely spiral further. So, stay calm and use a soothing voice.

An action to reduce anxiety is to recognize and praise small accomplishments, especially things that may have given your child trouble in the past. Celebrate the little successes. Praise your child for being brave and facing the challenge in front of her.

Make sure you have reasonable expectations as to what your child can and cannot do right now. She may require more help than in the past or is usual for her age. Try not to punish negative behavior or regressions. While your child might have been able to do something easily today, tomorrow that same skill may not be obtainable. Know that these regressions do and will happen.

Big feelings may come with anxiety. It is important that you help your child understand that feelings are normal and teach her how to express her feelings verbally as much as possible. Ask questions to help your child understand the root cause of her feelings. She may not be able to express it or even understand it.

Another thing you can do is to break down big tasks into smaller steps and focus on taking it one step at a time. If your child is too worried to even get started, ask her, "What's the worst thing that can happen?" Perhaps helping her to understand that the worst thing isn't so bad may help her take that first step.

Medicine/Supplements

Taking medicine or supplements can be challenging for some children, especially when it involves swallowing lots of them. If you can teach your child to swallow pills, it will help ease this daily process.

The best method that I found to help teach my children to swallow pills was created and developed by Professor Bonnie Kaplan, in conjunction with the University of Calgary and the Alberta Children's Hospital Research

Institute. She has an instructional video listed in the resource section of this book. It involves teaching your child five different ways to swallow and uses candy increasing in size to help her learn how in a comfortable way. When I told my daughters that they would get candy every day for two weeks for learning to swallow them, they were in!

If your child still has difficulty swallowing due to the taste of the pills, you may want to explore having her take them with different beverages that mask the taste. This could be juice, iced tea or even chocolate milk. Your child might be open to explore if she is given the power to select a few beverage options to try.

For liquid medicines that your child doesn't like the taste of or doesn't want to take, try mixing it into applesauce, pudding, ice cream or smoothies. Ask your child what the medicine could be mixed into. Perhaps they have a few different ideas and when a child has more control of the process, she is more likely to agree to try.

Compounding medicine can be another option for children who are unable to swallow pills. In drug compounding, a special pharmacy will combine, mix or alter two or more drug ingredients to create a medication tailored to the needs of an individual patient. Compounded drugs are not approved by the Food and Drug Administration (FDA). This means the FDA does not verify the safety or effectiveness of compounded drugs. Therefore, it is very important to find a good compounding pharmacy to work with.

Some children have difficulty swallowing liquids due to their taste or smell. The pharmacist can also help identify good flavors to mask the medicinal taste so your child will tolerate it.

When my daughter didn't like the smell or taste of a supplement that could not be taken with food, I purchased empty, clear capsules and put the drops of liquid into the capsule, which she would then swallow. This solved her problem and removed a challenge from our daily dosing. These empty capsules can be purchased online and at select grocery stores. You'll just need to be aware of the different capsule size options.

This solution may also be used for unpleasant-tasting antibiotic caplets or tablets. When my daughter had to take a caplet but did not like the taste, I cut it in half and put it in the capsule for her to swallow. This removed the challenge and helped her get it down.

When filling medications, you may want to pay attention to the brand names. Different brands have different colors and tastes, which can create challenges for our children. One P/P mom suggests asking the pharmacists before filling the prescription which brand they have on hand to avoid wasting money and time.

A few parents have shared that their child will no longer willingly take medicine due to a fear of it being poisoned. If this is the case, see if you can safely take the medicine once to show them it is not poisonous to them. This may work better with supplements or homeopathy; however, do ask your physician if it is a possibility.

School

Getting out the door, especially in the morning for school, can be hard. One therapist we worked with suggested having my daughter take her shower at night and wear her school clothes to bed. This eliminated the overwhelming task of selecting an outfit first thing in the morning and shortened our morning routine. This was especially helpful when she was experiencing sleep issues.

Another trick we learned was to keep her toothbrush, toothpaste, washcloth and facial soap in the bathroom closest to the front door. This way she could wash and brush on her way out and not get side-tracked.

We also struggled to get out the door on time with the medicine my daughter had to take. I literally gave them to her in the parking lot at school before dropping her off. This kept her from lingering when she was excited to get into school. Once she was in front of the school, taking the medicine would go much faster.

At first, my daughter didn't want to go to school because of separation anxiety. To help her deal with those moments of sadness during the day, she brought a picture of us with her to school. Whenever she was sad and missing me, she took it out of her bag to look at. She also brought a small comfort item with her. Some children are not able to attend school when dealing with P/P, but this tip might help if your child is just on the edge of making it through.

One friend had a son who would say at night that he would go to school the next day, but in the morning his anxiety would take over and keep him from attending. To address this constant struggle, her husband encouraged their son to record a message to himself at night reminding himself of all the reasons why he wanted to go to school. It worked! He went, at least for a few more days.

Bribery is never out of the question. One time, I made a deal with my daughter that I would paint a pink heart on my cheek and wear it to drop-off if she could make it out the door on time that morning. That offer motivated her. I rocked the biggest, brightest pink heart on my cheek that day and had a good laugh. However, be careful with bribery when a child can't go because of OCD or anxiety, as not getting the prize can be even more upsetting on top of not being able to go to school.

School pick-up can be rough. Your child may have held it together all day long and now that you are physically present, she might completely fall apart, as you are her safe space. While understandable, it can be incredibly difficult to manage, especially when trying to drive home. As a result, be sure to build in time between the end of the school day and wherever you are going. Have a planned place to pull over, perhaps the parking lot, to hang out for a while.

The frontal lobe of the brain is responsible for executive functioning, including impulse control, and it does not fully develop until a person is 25 years old. Some suggest that having protein can help optimize brain function and regulate brain activity. As a result, I would always have a protein-based snack available for after school pickup. She would start eating it the minute she got in the car. We even tried giving her an extra snack in her backpack to eat before she left the classroom at the end of the day. Did it help? I think so. It was absolutely worth trying and there was no downside. She needed an after-school snack anyway.

Homework refusal can also be a challenge. If necessary, reach out to the school and see if you can get an accommodation or exemption. Perhaps they need unlimited time to complete the homework to reduce anxiety. Or maybe they could get approval to type out homework instead of writing it. At the end of the day, a few months without any homework likely won't hurt anyone. Many research studies have shown homework to be somewhat ineffective anyway.

Partnering with the teacher and brainstorming ways to help your child attend may also be helpful. One friend had a son who had been out for a while and was hesitant to return. The teacher suggested visiting the classroom after school hours, so it would be less overwhelming on the first day back.

While these tips may help your child be able to attend school, please know that it is very common for P/P children to need a break from the brick-and-mortar school setting for numerous reasons. Forcing them to attend, when they are not able, may backfire and make things even worse. Listen to your child and her individual needs and partner with her to find the method for education at the moment. Many P/P children may take time off and then return and thrive. So, if these tips don't work for your child, don't fret.

Sensory Issues

P/P may cause significant sensory issues that may affect your child's ability to wear clothing and shoes. This can hinder her ability to leave the house. To manage this frustrating situation, I recommend buying multiple pairs of the same socks, pants, shirts, etc. that your child will wear. Buy clothes that are tagless or even cut the tags out. A quick internet search will also reveal sensory-friendly clothing that is soft and seamless.

Weighted blankets are also a great way to help soothe your child during the day or calm them for sleep at night. For daytime, there are smaller lap-sized blankets. The usual way of determining the weight of the blanket for your child is by calculating 10 percent of her overall body weight plus a pound or two. Some kids may crave more weight and their blanket may be closer to 20 percent. These blankets can be purchased online. Check the blanket's minimum age and weight to ensure a proper fit. Also, check the filler type to ensure your child won't get too hot.

One mom I spoke with shared that brushing therapy (Wilbarger Protocol) can be very helpful for sensory issues. It involves brushing the body with a small, soft surgical brush for a few minutes throughout the day. It is like a deep pressure massage that is reported to decrease sensory defensiveness and anxiety. If you think that your child would benefit from brushing, you'll want to seek guidance from an occupational therapist.

Feeling wet in the vaginal area is a very common sensory issue for girls. Some children will stay in the bathroom wiping nonstop as a result. One trick that helped my daughter is to have her wear a panty liner. It would remove the feeling of moisture and give her more confidence and comfort.

Some children experience issues with loud noises. To help them overcome this challenge, consider getting a pair of noise-canceling headphones. From the blender in the kitchen to the hand dryer in public restrooms, this will help keep things a little more manageable.

Brushing teeth seems to be another issue that many children deal with. There are a few tricks you can explore here. First, you can try altering the type of toothbrush to an electric from a manual (if you don't already have one) as some dentists suggest that the electric toothbrush does a better job getting rid of plaque.

If your child doesn't want to brush, there are phone apps that you can download that encourage brushing. The child starts brushing and when the timer is up, she will be rewarded with virtual stickers.

Another strategy is to make it a game! Hide a toy and have your child brush around the house while she looks for it. Or you could time how long it takes her to brush in each room of the house.

One friend would brush her dog's teeth at the same time as her child would brush. This would provide a great distraction for her child and make it less stressful.

If all else fails, there are some therapeutic mouthwashes that can be prescribed by a dentist that are more effective than over-the-counter mouthwashes.

Sleep

A lack of sleep (for the child as well as the parent) is one of the worst symptoms of these diseases as they impact everyone's ability to deal with all other symptoms!

One thing that we have found helpful over the years is establishing a consistent bedtime routine. Set clear expectations on when that routine will start and what it will involve. Give 15-minute, 10-minute and 5-minute countdown warnings before it's time to get in bed.

Another tip is to incorporate restorative yoga. Restorative yoga involves poses that calm and reset the body and mind to prepare your body for relaxation. As I mentioned in Chapter 7, restorative yoga is good for you as well as your child. A 10-minute session seems like a good amount of time for my kids to decompress, though some kids may need more or less. There are many free apps available to download.

Once in bed, it can be helpful to listen to a soothing sleep or calming meditation for 10 to 20 minutes. Often, I sit or lie down next to them. Again, there are many apps available, some even for free.

While yoga and meditation may help, they alone don't always do the trick. You may want to explore supplements to aid in sleep, such as melatonin, CBD products, l'theanine or a combination.

According to the American Academy of Pediatrics, "melatonin is a natural, hormone-like substance produced by an area in the brain called the pineal gland. It is released naturally at night and tells the body it's time to sleep." Its use is not regulated by the FDA or approved for that purpose. Since there are no specific guidelines on melatonin, work with your physician to determine the appropriate dosage for your child.

Charlotte's Web, a pioneer in the CBD industry since 2012, makes an effective sleep gummy that combines melatonin and CBD. It's best to give melatonin and/or CBD 30 minutes before bedtime for a better night's sleep.

Another tip is to communicate with your spouse or partner about who is responsible for what at bedtime. Who is overseeing the bedtime routine? Who is tucking the child in? You also may want to split up the night so that one person is on call for the first half of the night and the other person for the second half, or even rotate nights. This may help you both get a decent amount of sleep over the course of a week.

If your child has a strong preference for which parent she would like to put her to bed, this can complicate your plan. If you are that parent, make sure you communicate with your partner on how he or she can be supportive during that time, such as doing other things around the house like dishes or laundry, and be sure to acknowledge that the preference is nothing personal.

Rages/Tantrums

Sometimes the rages or tantrums can be absolutely brutal and dangerous. There are a few things you may want to experiment with to make them safer for everyone involved.

Remove all objects that can be dangerous from your child's room, including glass or breakable items and items of sentimental value. When your child is beginning an episodic rage at home, redirect the child to her room so that if she starts throwing objects you can limit the physical damage done to items and people.

Depending upon the severity of your child's tantrums or rages, you may want to consider putting away any dangerous objects throughout the house. While we didn't have to put away our kitchen knives, I did speak with a few families who needed to lock them away in a secure cabinet for a while.

If your child's rage involves hitting or biting, you might want to separate any other children in the home during this time. The primary focus is to keep everyone safe.

When your child is in an out-of-control rage, you can gently but firmly hold her to prevent her from harming herself or others. The use of physical intervention can be used in an emergency when your child is posing an immediate danger to herself or others. Physical restraint should be used only as a last resort when all other attempts to calm your child's escalating behavior have been tried and have failed.

* * *

P/P is a journey that is filled with ups and downs. It is a puzzle that requires putting lots of pieces together: getting a proper diagnosis, finding the best treatment, reframing expectations, establishing support systems and embracing self-care. Hopefully this survival guide has given you the tools and confidence you and your family need to tackle this illness while maintaining your sanity. Know that you are not alone. There are thousands of parents out there fighting your same battle. This book is just the beginning. The more knowledge you have, the more empowered and successful you will be in helping your child throughout the healing process.

Chapter 9: Additional Resources

P/P Websites/Blogs

- Aspire Care (www.aspire.com)
- National Institute of Mental Health (www.nimh.nih.gov/health/publications/pandas/index.shtml)
- PANDAS Network (www.pandasnetwork.org)
- PANDAS Physicians Network (www.pandasppn.org)
- Panslife.com (www.panslife.com)
- Pediatric Research and Advocacy Initiative (PRAI) (www.praikids.org)
- The Foundation for Children with Neuroimmune Disorders (www.neuroimmune.org)

Association Presentations

- Dr. M. Elizabeth Latimer, MD, *The Spectrum of PANDAS: One Size Does Not Fit All,* New England PANS/PANDAS Parent Association Conference, November 2013 (https://youtu.be/suI6icFfIag)

- Dr. Susan E. Swedo, MD, PANDAS/PANS Standards of Care Summit, October 4, 2018 (https://youtu.be/CqjTIyW-xYg)

P/P-Friendly Practitioners

- PANDAS Physicians Network's searchable practitioner database (www.pandasppn.org/practitioners/)

Documentaries

- *My Kid Is Not Crazy* (www.mykidisnotcrazy.com)
- *Our PANS Story* (https://youtu.be/H2zB1ZRcuh8)
- *PANS/PANDAS: A Survivor's Story* (https://youtu.be/6HRpARojZnU)
- *A Childhood Mystery: PANDAS and PANS Disorder* (www.pbs.org/video/pandaspans-lvnbrl/)
- *Stolen Childhood* (https://youtu.be/Cprp-zhkDCM)

Books for Adults

- *A Parents' Guide to PANDAS, PANS, and Related Neuroimmune Disorders*. Doran, Amabile, et al., Jessica Kingsley Publishers, 2019.
- *Brain Under Attack: A Resource for Parents and Caregivers of Children with PANS, PANDAS, and Autoimmune Encephalitis*. Lambert, Beth et. al., Answers Publications, 2018.

- *Childhood Interrupted: The Complete Guide to PANDAS and PANS*. Maloney, Beth Alison. CreateSpace Independent Publishing Platform, 2013.
- *PANDAS and PANS in School Settings*. Doran, Patricia Rice. Jessica Kingsley Publishers, 2016.
- *PANDAS: Reaching Out - A Natural and Homeopathic Approach*. Bentley, Grant. CreateSpace Independent Publishing Platform, 2016.
- *PANS, CANS, and Automobiles: A Comprehensive Reference Guide for Helping Students with PANDAS and PANS*. Greene, Jamie Candelaria. First Edition Design Publishing, 2016.
- *Saving Sammy: A Mother's Fight to Cure Her Son's OCD*. Maloney, Beth Alison. Broadway Books, 2010.
- *Shadow Syndromes: Shining a Light on PANS and Other Inflammation Based Illnesses Plaguing Today's Youth*. Any Mom®. CreateSpace Independent Publishing Platform, 2017.
- *What Happened to My Child?: A Mother's Courageous Journey to Save Her Son*. Korbmacher, Heather. Author Academy Elite, 2019.
- *Wrestling Hurricanes*. Haines, Tiffany. Morgan James Faith Publisher, 2021.

Books for Children

- *In A Pickle Over PANDAS*. Weiss, Melanie S. First Edition Design Publishing. 2015.
- *My Story About PANS/PANDAS*. Bassman Ross, Keri and Avery, Dr. Rachel. Ross Consulting, 2019.
- *PANS/PANDAS Strength - Hope - Understanding: A Picture Book for Children, Family, & Educators*. Gushansky, Suzann. CreateSpace Independent Publishing Platform, 2018.
- *Super Sam and the Battle Against PANS/PANDAS*. Wells, Dr. Lindsey. Lindsey Wells ND, LLC, 2021.

Facebook Groups (National Groups)

- Homeopathy for PANS & PANDAS
- Homeschooling PANDAS
- Low Dose Immune Therapy for AUTISM, PANDAS, PANS and Its Co-infections
- P.A.N.D.A.S. Network
- PANDAS Parents
- PANDAS – Pediatric Autoimmune Neuropsychiatric Disorder Associated w/Strep
- PANDAS Syndrome Support Group
- PANDAS/PANS Autoimmune Encephalitis Recovery
- PANDAS Parents IVIG Information Sharing
- PANS/PANDAS Parent Support

- PANDAS/PANS Parent Stress Relief Group
- PANDAS & PANS Advocacy in Schools
- PARENTS of CHILDREN with PANDAS/PANS/LYME/TICK-BORNE DISEASES
- The PANS Party Project
- Unschooling, Relaxed Homeschooling, Life Learning PANDAS/PANS

Lyme Disease & Co-infections

- Global Lyme Alliance (www.globallymealliance.org)
- International Lyme and Associated Disease Society (www.ilads.org)

School Resources

- PANDAS Network – school page (www.pandasnetwork.org/school)
- New England PANS/PANDAS – school page (www.nepans.org/school-resources.html)
- PANDAS Physicians Network – school page (www.pandasppn.org/school)
- Family Unschooling Network (www.unschooling.org)

Post-Traumatic Stress Disorder (PTSD)

- American Psychiatric Association (www.psychiatry.org/patients-families/ptsd/what-is-ptsd)
- Mayo Clinic (www.mayoclinic.org/diseases-conditions/post-traumatic-stress-disorder/symptoms-causes/syc-20355967)
- National Institute of Mental Health (www.nimh.nih.gov/health/topics/post-traumatic-stress-disorder-ptsd/index.shtml)

Swallowing Pills

- Dr. Bonnie J Kaplan, *Better Than a Spoonful of Sugar: How to Swallow Pills.* October 9, 2019 (https://bonniejkaplan.com/how-to-swallow-pills)

Alternative Treatment Options

- American Institute of Homeopathy (www.homeopathyusa.org)
- The Institute for Functional Medicine (www.ifm.org)

Acknowledgements

My younger P/P daughter recently published her first book at age 11. If you had told me seven years ago this would be possible, I would not have believed you. If you had told me seven years ago that she would inspire me to write my own book, I would have laughed.

I would like to thank both of my daughters for teaching me more about myself in the past seven years than I had learned in the previous 39. I admire their strength and resilience. They are my heroes. Thank you, girls, for sharing our story to benefit others. While none of us wanted to be on this journey, I'm grateful for the silver linings our family has gained along the way.

I would also like to thank my husband for his unconditional love and partnership, as well as his contributions to this book. I would have drowned if it were not for him. There is no one else I'd rather be with to face this difficult and relentless illness. P/P continues to bring us together and make us stronger as a couple.

Thank you does not seem like enough when it comes to the contributions of my good friend, fellow P/P mom and amazing editor, Melissa Nolan. This book rose to a whole new level with your guidance. Thank you for spending hours with me every Monday night to dissect each paragraph, sentence and word in this book. Our friendship is my silver lining for which I am eternally grateful.

This journey would have been far longer if it weren't for my mother-in-law, Ada Marcus, who made the connection between our child's symptoms and that of her friend's grandson and suggested a Lyme test. Another thank you to Rachel Leslie of Whole Soul Counseling in Connecticut. She is the daughter of my mother-in-law's friend who educated us on P/P and Lyme disease, recommended local doctors who treat these illnesses, and suggested tests to request from those doctors. Rachel immediately set us on the right path, and we are incredibly grateful.

Thank you to Dr. Philip G. Kazlow in the Gastroenterology department at Colombia University's Department of Pediatrics for performing the Lyme test for our younger daughter while helping us explore her gastrointestinal issues. Encouraging us to find the right doctor to further evaluate the inconclusive Lyme test result was a critical step in our journey.

A big thank you goes out to our outstanding medical support, Dr. Denis Bouboulis of Advanced Allergy

Immunology & Asthma PC, and Jana Roso, MSN, RN, CPNP, MAPS Fellow of Alive and Well, who have saved our children with their knowledge, understanding and effective treatment approaches for PANDAS, PANS, Lyme and other tickborne illnesses. Thank you both for reviewing this book and providing additional content and support.

This book would not have been complete if it weren't for the contributions of others. Thank you to Dr. Sarah Griesemer, Ph.D., of Psychology Center of Austin, for your valuable advice for parents based on your years of professional experience.

A big thank you is in order for fellow P/P parents for their contributions, including Robyn Herbert, Jessica Gavin, Kelly Oliver and Melissa Stein. In addition, the chapter on the kid's perspective could not have been written without the bravery of the many children who shared their thoughts and stories for the benefit of others.

Lastly, the P/P community on social media has been instrumental with helping to provide support and guidance. I can't take credit for all the tips and tricks in this book, as many were passed along from other parents on this journey.

Index

About the Author

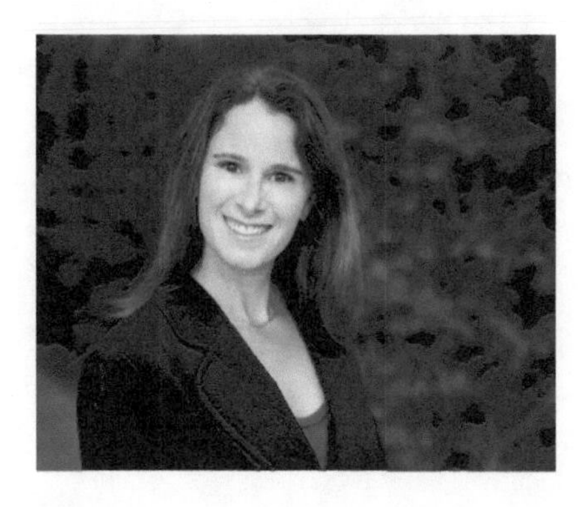

Deborah Marcus has been a mom of two children with PANDAS/PANS, Lyme disease and other tickborne illnesses since 2014, and has since guided many families dealing with these illnesses. *The Parent's Survival Guide to PANDAS/PANS* is her first book, which was written with the sole purpose of expanding her reach and support to others in this growing community.

Deb is an energetic, enthusiastic and optimistic business consultant. She earned her BA from Syracuse University and her MBA from The University of North Carolina at Chapel Hill. She lives in Austin, TX, with her husband and two daughters and enjoys spending time with family and friends, walking their rescue dog, Laci, and relieving stress through indoor spinning, weightlifting, yoga and meditation.

Made in United States
Troutdale, OR
11/16/2023

14638265R00090